DEPARTMENT OF HEALTH AND SOCIAL SECURITY

Prevention and Health: Avoiding Heart Attacks

London: Her Majesty's Stationery Office

ISBN 0 11 320771 9

Contents

Tables

Figures

Foreword

Coronary heart disease is a killer. In 1978 it accounted for almost 185,000 deaths in the United Kingdom! It can affect both men and women, but for middle aged men it is by far the most important single cause of death in the UK. It is also a major cause of debilitating sickness. Prevention of coronary heart disease has therefore a vital role to play in reducing human suffering and also in relieving the burden on the National Health Service

This booklet on coronary heart disease is one of a series issued by our Departments on 'Prevention and Health'. It explains the nature of the disease and the size of the problem. It looks at various factors which put people at greater risk of getting the disease. Some of the evidence is incomplete or even conflicting and, where this is so, it is discussed frankly. But where the evidence is conclusive, clear advice is given on how the risk of getting a heart attack can be reduced.

The booklet should be particularly useful to people working in the health, social and education services, including teachers and health education officers. But we hope that it will also provide the individual reader with the information needed to judge the implications for his or her own life-style and to consider what he or she should do to avoid a heart attack.

NORMAN FOWLER
Secretary of State for Social Services

GEORGE YOUNGER
Secretary of State for Scotland

NICHOLAS EDWARDS
Secretary of State for Wales

JAMES PRIOR
Secretary of State for Northern Ireland

CHAPTER I '....suddenly....'

One day recently an announcement appeared in the obituary columns of the *Liverpool Morning Post* which read:

> 'SMITH, on Feb 16, suddenly, John Bernard ("JB") Smith of 236 Henley Street, dearly loved husband of Mary and father of Richard and Susan. Funeral arrangements later.'

A small paragraph in the evening paper, the *Liverpool Evening Sketch,* the previous day had given some more information.

> '*Death of Salesman*: Mr John Bernard Smith, 41, of Henley Street, was found slumped over his desk at home yesterday. Mr Smith, a sales representative, was dead on arrival at Sefton General Hospital. He leaves a widow and two young children. The coroner has been informed.'

The coroner ordered an autopsy and the pathologist found that John Bernard Smith had died of coronary heart disease.

The details have been changed but the story is all too familiar and might have appeared in any one of a hundred local newspapers. Sometimes, when the dead person is a politician, a well-known actor or a famous pop-star, the news may even flash for a day or two across the national press. It is the tale of a life cut down in its prime, of death striking swiftly and unexpectedly, often just as a person is coming to assume increasing responsibilities towards his family and his job.

What is coronary heart disease?

Is it really more common than it used to be?

Why is it usually men who appear to be hit by it? Are women somehow immune?

What causes the disease and is it possible to prevent it?

These are the questions which this booklet is concerned to examine and if possible to answer. A fairly straightforward reply can be given to some of the questions but to others we simply have no clear answer. The best that can be done is to set out the evidence and let the reader judge. In reaching his decision he will bear in mind that what is at stake could be, quite literally, a matter of life or death. For those who have already suffered a heart attack the advice given is of particular importance.

For an understanding of the problem some background knowledge is needed of the way the heart works and of some of the things that can go wrong—matters dealt with in Chapter II.

In dealing with a specialised subject of any kind technical terms cannot be avoided, and this subject is no exception. As they arise technical terms are explained but to help the reader coming across them anew these terms have also been brought together in a glossary at the end of the booklet. A list for further reading—the literature is enormous and growing—is also included.

CHAPTER II What is coronary heart disease?

In everyday speech such phrases as 'He had a coronary' or 'He died of a heart attack' are often used and translated into medical terms these almost always imply coronary heart disease. To understand something of the disease, its causes and its prevention, requires some basic knowledge of the heart and how it works.

How the heart works

In strictly mechanical terms the heart (Fig. 1) is nothing more than a pump. Its job is to ensure the continuous and uninterrupted circulation of blood so that every living cell in the body, however remote from the centre, may be kept supplied with oxygen, food, and the other chemical substances needed to maintain life. The wall of the heart consists mainly of a special type of muscle, called myocardium, arranged in an intricate pattern of rings and spirals. By contracting, the myocardium expels the blood from the chambers of the heart, and one-way valves ensure that the blood is propelled onwards. In a resting adult, the heart muscle contracts (ie the heart beats) about 60 times per minute. In a day it pumps about 7000 litres (over 7 tons) of blood. Physical activity, anger or other strong emotion increases both the rate of the heart beat and also the amount expelled at each beat, the circulation of blood being greatly accelerated.

The heart is really a double pump (Fig. 1). Blood from the left main chamber (left ventricle) of the heart is expelled into the main artery (the aorta) which leads off into branches supplying blood to all parts of the body. Having yielded up its oxygen the blood returns by veins to the right side of the heart. From there it is pumped by the right ventricle into the pulmonary artery and passes through the lungs where it picks up a fresh load of oxygen. The oxygenated blood then returns by the pulmonary vein to the left side of the heart, and is expelled into the aorta, thus completing the circulation.

In order to do the work demanded of it, the myocardium itself, just like any other tissue, has to be supplied with oxygen and nutrients. Not surprisingly,

Fig. 1.   The heart and general circulation. The heart consists of two chambers —
an atrium and a muscular ventricle — on each side. The flaps between
each atrium and ventricle and at the origins of the aorta and pulmonary
artery are one-way valves.

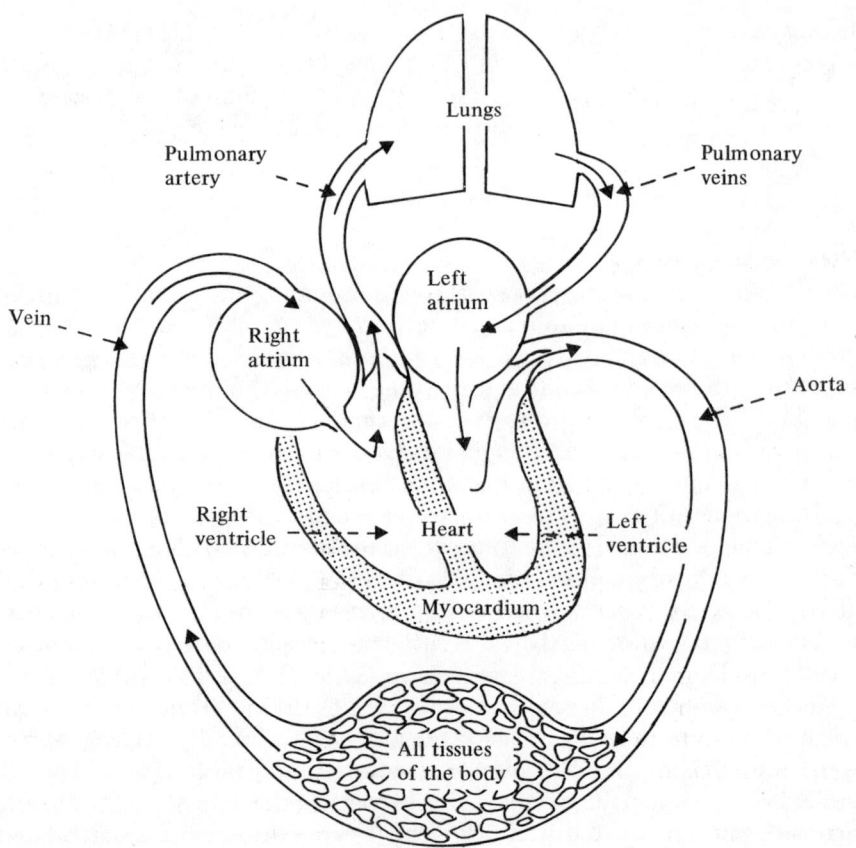

therefore, the very first branches to lead off from the aorta are the two coronary arteries, which supply blood to the heart muscle (Fig. 2).

Coronary heart disease

Anything which interferes seriously with the normal flow of blood through the coronary arteries impairs the nutrition of the myocardium and reduces the efficiency of the heart as a pump. By far the most important cause of reduced coronary blood flow is *atheroma* of the coronary arteries. This consists of patches of thickening of the walls of the coronary arteries with consequent narrowing of the bore of the arteries, the lumen. The patches consist partly of deposits of lipids (fatty materials, including cholesterol—see later) and partly of dense scar tissue. There may be many such patches; they form and grow slowly and so are increasingly common and large in middle and old age. By severely narrowing the lumen of coronary arteries, atheroma can reduce considerably the blood supply to the myocardium. *Thrombosis* (formation of a blood clot) is liable to occur over a patch of atheroma and completely block the artery.

These changes in the coronary arteries give rise to three forms of coronary heart disease—*sudden death*, an 'acute heart attack' (*myocardial infarction*) and *angina pectoris* ('angina').

Sudden death can result from severe coronary artery atheroma alone or with superadded thrombosis. Coronary heart disease is the major cause of sudden death apart from injury.

The second form of the disease, an acute heart attack or myocardial infarction, results from loss of the blood supply to part of the myocardium, usually due to blockage of a coronary artery by thrombosis (Fig. 2). The deprived patch of myocardium stops contracting and dies, eventually to be replaced by a scar if the patient survives. Clinically, the acute heart attack is usually accompanied by severe chest pain which resembles the pain of angina (see below) but is more persistent, continuing for some hours or even days.

The third form of the disease, angina, might be described as 'the cry of the heart for oxygen'. It takes the form of a severe pain in the chest, sometimes spreading up into the neck or down the arms. It is generally brought on by exertion particularly in cold weather or when the heart is loaded with extra work after a heavy meal, and is usually relieved quickly by resting. The word angina comes from the Latin for strangling or gripping hard, and that is how people with angina often describe the sensation. Angina usually follows narrowing of the coronary arteries by atheroma but may occur rarely without pre-existing atheroma.

By the age of 40, nearly all men and many women in this country have some patches of atheroma on the coronary arteries, but the patches are often too

Fig. 2. Diagram of the ventricles of the heart, showing the two coronary arteries, which are branches of the aorta. Obstruction of an artery deprives part of the myocardium of blood supply. If complete, the obstruction causes an infarct (shaded area); if incomplete (due to atheroma), angina may result.

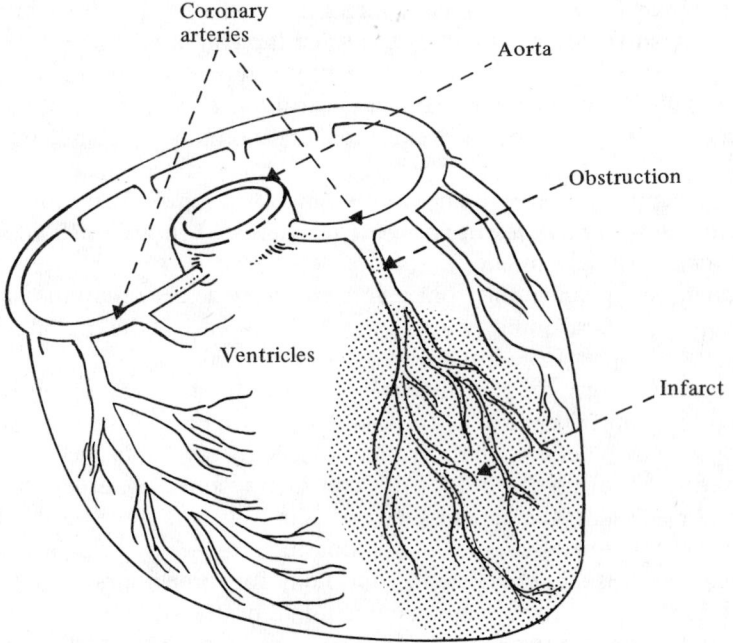

small to interfere seriously with the blood supply to the heart, and are detected only at post-mortem examination of people dying of other causes. Coronary heart disease develops only in individuals with large patches of atheroma or with superadded thrombosis. There is no simple method of detecting symptomless coronary artery atheroma.

The amount of oxygen the heart must have at any time depends on the amount of work it is being called upon to perform, and on the efficiency with which it is performing that work. One result of being 'in training' is that the efficiency of the heart's action is improved so that it is capable of taking on a given work-load with less expenditure of effort and thus with less demand for oxygen. But in all healthy people the heart has in any case a considerable reserve capacity and the coronary circulation, if called upon to do so, can provide the myocardium with several times the volume of blood per minute that it delivers when the person is at rest. As we grow older the reserve capacity falls off, partly because of the development of atheroma, and partly because the coronary arteries lose their elasticity and therefore their potential for increasing the blood flow to the heart muscle. How much oxygen a given volume of blood can carry depends on how much haemoglobin (the substance in red blood cells which carries oxygen) is in that volume of blood. Sometimes there is not enough haemoglobin, as in anaemia or after a severe hae-morrhage. Oxygen demand is then more likely to exceed supply and angina may result.

CHAPTER III The size of the problem

In discussing the problem of coronary heart disease it is important to determine as far as possible whether this is a new disease or an old one that has suddenly become more frequent. But in either case there has to be a reason and if we knew the reason then perhaps we could do something about it.

A short history

The most alarming form of the disease—sudden death—is certainly not new. Pliny the Elder, the Roman historian, tells of a senator of ancient Rome who collapsed and died on his way out of the Senate where he had just delivered a powerful speech. He also recounts the case of a nobleman who died suddenly while visiting a certain dancer, reputed to be the most famous beauty of her day (the same fate apparently befell another gentleman in her company). Angina, another form of the disease, has been known at least from the early years of the eighteenth century. John Hunter, the Scot who came to London and transformed surgery into a science, suffered greatly from angina as he grew older. He used to say that his life was in the hands of any scoundrel who chose to annoy him. When he died in 1793 during a prolonged attack brought on after a meeting, his one-time pupil and colleague, Edward Jenner of smallpox vaccination fame, correctly predicted that at the autopsy the coronary arteries would be found to be grossly diseased.

Evidently, therefore, coronary heart disease cannot be regarded as new. What can be said is that it has become very much more common in recent times. In the past some people tried to argue that the disease itself had not increased much in incidence but that it was being diagnosed more often, especially since the introduction of the electrocardiograph (an instrument which measures changes in the electrical activity of the heart during the cycle of contraction) in the period between the two world wars. At best, the argument could only partially explain why, according to the records, the disease has become so much more frequent than it used to be. In his day Sir William Osler was the most eminent physician on either side of the Atlantic, and yet in his classic lectures on heart disease delivered in London in 1910 he could recall seeing only a few score cases of coronary heart disease in the course of a long and busy professional career.

Coronary heart disease in the UK today

Whatever the arguments in the past, the consensus today is that the prevalence of coronary heart disease has increased greatly over the last half-century. The death rates for the United Kingdom are shown in Figure 3. It is clear from these that the rate for men is higher than for women, and that the rate for both sexes increases with age.

The extent of the change that has taken place in the death rates in the United Kingdom in the last thirty years is illustrated in Figure 4 (a, b, and c). The average of the rates for the years 1950-52 has been taken as 100 in each Figure and the curves show the change over the period up to 1977 in England and Wales, Scotland and Northern Ireland, for males and females in three main age groups. Significantly —

the changes in the rates for males have been much more marked than those for females;

the increase in the rates for males has been most marked in the youngest age group, 35-44 years, and in this age group in England and Wales the death rate doubled in the 15 years from 1950-65;

there is a suggestion that the rate in this youngest group has started to fall in the last few years, at least in England and Wales and in Scotland;

from about 1960 onwards the rates among females aged 35-44 years have risen sharply in England and Wales, though not in Scotland and Northern Ireland.

As a cause of death in the United Kingdom the importance of coronary heart disease may be judged from Figure 5 which shows (by sex and age group) both the number of deaths from the disease in 1978, and the proportion of all deaths that this represents. With increasing age the numbers of deaths due to the disease increase rapidly, and so too does its relative importance compared with other causes of death. Thus, in the 45-54 age group it accounts for 2 out of every 5 male deaths. *Coronary heart disease is by far the most important single cause of death among middle-aged men in this country.*

But coronary heart disease is an important cause of sickness as well as of death. Between 1966 and 1975 hospital admission rates went up for both men and women aged between 35 and 64 years, but the rates for men were much higher throughout. During 1975 nearly 10,000 hospital beds were in constant use every day in the United Kingdom for the care of patients with coronary heart disease. While most of these patients would have been elderly, over 3000 beds were being occupied by patients under 65. The story is the same outside

Fig. 3.   Death rate per 100,000 population from coronary heart disease* in
United Kingdom, 1978

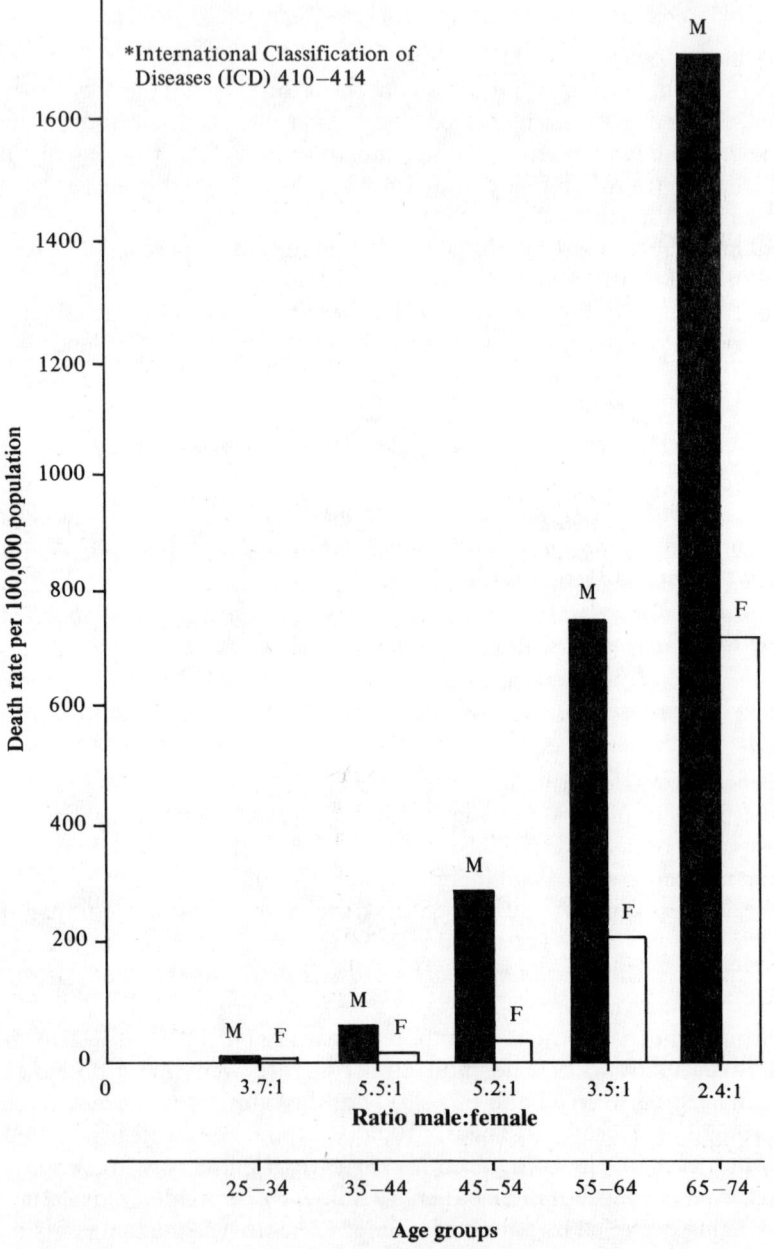

hospital. In a recent survey of the work of general practitioners in England and Wales it was found that between 30 and 40 of every 1000 men aged 45 to 64 saw their doctor each year on account of coronary heart disease.

It is also a major cause of absence from work: in 1975 $27\frac{1}{2}$ million working days were lost in the United Kingdom because of coronary heart disease, or heart conditions associated with high blood pressure.

International comparisons

This country is not alone in having experienced a rising trend over the past few decades in the death rate from coronary heart disease, particularly among men in middle life. In the United States, for instance, the overall death rate from coronary heart disease increased by nearly 50 per cent between 1940 and 1960. Large increases were recorded among older men in several other countries. However, the recent figures from the World Health Organisation show that the death rate has begun to go down again in the United States and a number of other countries (though not in England and Wales, where as Figure 4(a) shows, it has remained fairly constant for the last ten years). In the United States the death rate for men and women actually declined by 27 per cent between 1968 and 1976! It is difficult to show precise causes for this dramatic change in the United States; it has been suggested that greater public awareness in recent years of the dangers of cigarette smoking, over-eating, lack of exercise and high blood pressure may well have something to do with it. But the trend is first discernible about the same time that the decline in adult male tobacco consumption begins.

Although similar trends are found in different countries, the impact of coronary heart disease nevertheless varies from one country to another. Figure 6 compares the rates of males and females in 24 countries up to the age of 74.* For men, the highest death rate is that of Finland; Northern Ireland and Scotland are close behind, and Wales too had a rate only slightly lower. Although the death rate in England was not as high as elsewhere in the United Kingdom, it was much higher than in Belgium, Germany and Switzerland. In every country the death rate among females was well below that for males: only in Israel did the death rate of women come near that of men. Coronary heart disease is an uncommon condition in the less developed countries of the world. Where people have not come into close contact with 'civilisation' it is virtually unknown.

---

* Different countries have different systems of compiling their statistics and these differences could affect the interpretation of the data. For example, the death rate in France may not be truly comparable with the rates in Britain or the Netherlands. The reservation does not apply with the same force to comparisons between countries within Scandinavia or within the United Kingdom.

Although Figure 6 shows the death rates and not the number of new cases of the disease, a World Heath Organisation study of twelve European cities in the early 1970s showed that national differences in the frequency of *attacks* of coronary heart disease corresponded closely with the differences in frequency of *deaths* from the disease.

Regional variations
Just as there are differences between countries, so too are there differences within individual countries in the number of new cases and the number of deaths from coronary heart disease. Thus, Figure 7 indicates the broad variation in death rate of men of middle age within the United Kingdom. The highest rate (West Central Scotland) was almost double the lowest (East Anglia). Similarly, variations have been often noted within Belgium, Canada, Finland and the United States.

How great is the danger of heart disease?
The study of European cities mentioned earlier allows us to estimate the chance of a 40 year old man having a heart attack.

Taking the highest recorded rate in each age group, one can calculate that of every 1000 men aged 40 who had not had a previous heart attack, about 200 or one in five will suffer at least one attack before the age of 65. Considerable though the problem certainly is, it is as well to keep it in some kind of proportion, and to remember that by the same token 4 men in 5 will escape the experience.

Fig. 4(a). Change in death rates of men and women in three age groups (from 35-64 years) from coronary heart disease[1] in England and Wales, 1950—1978 (3 year moving averages 1950—52 = 100%).

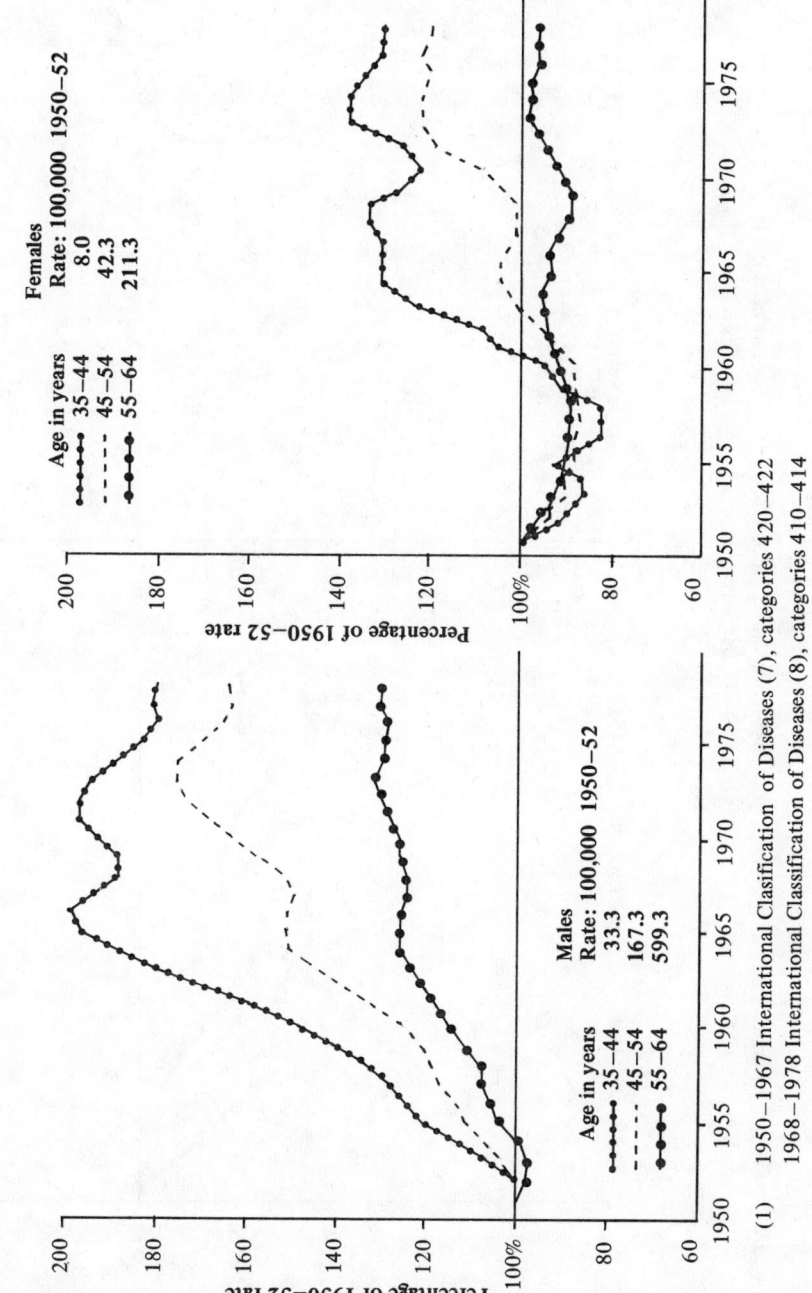

(1) 1950—1967 International Clasification of Diseases (7), categories 420—422

1968—1978 International Classification of Diseases (8), categories 410—414

Fig. 4(b).   Change in death rates of men and women in three age groups (from 35–64 years) from coronary heart disease[1] in Scotland, 1950–1978 (3 year moving averages 1950–52 = 100%).

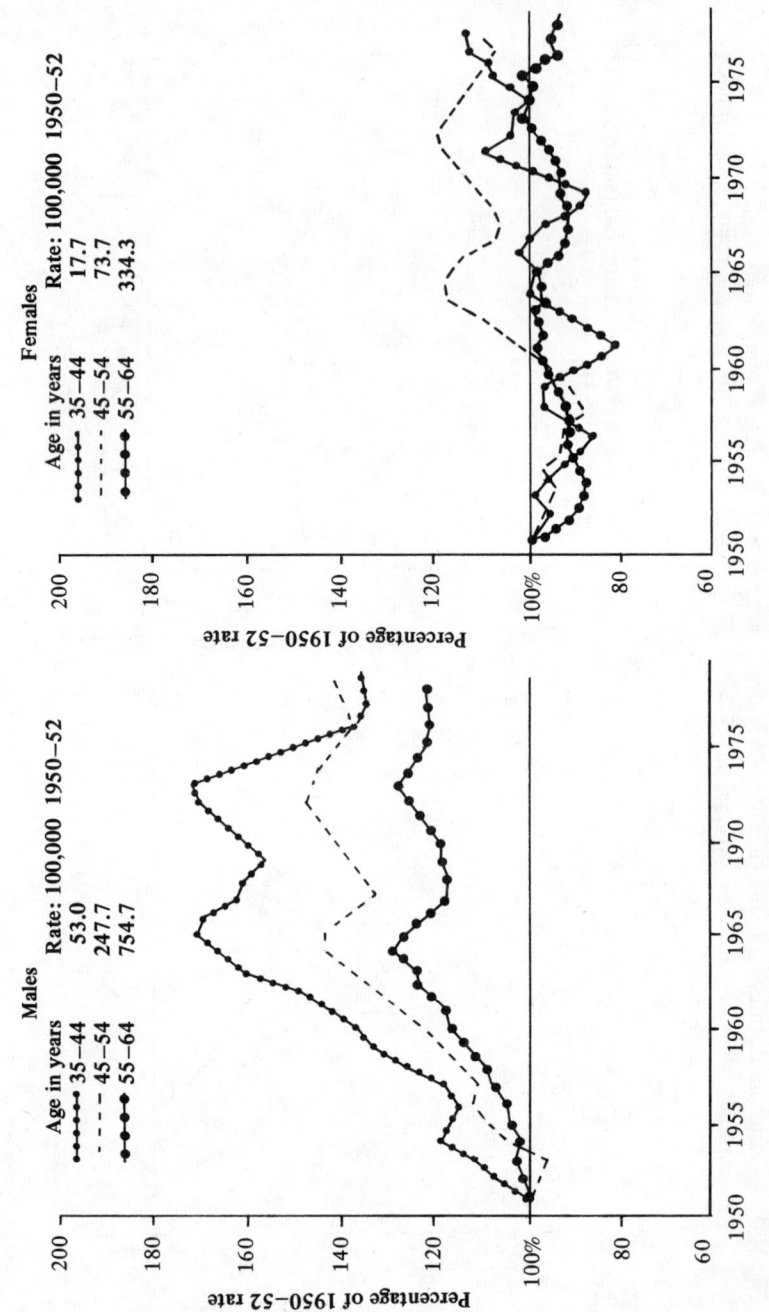

(1)   1950–1967 International Classification of Diseases (7), categories 420–422
1968–1978 International Classification of Diseases (8), categories 410–414

Fig. 4(c). Change in death rates of men and women in three age groups (from 35-64 years) from coronary heart disease[1] in Northern Ireland, 1950–1978 (3 year moving averages 1950–52 = 100%).

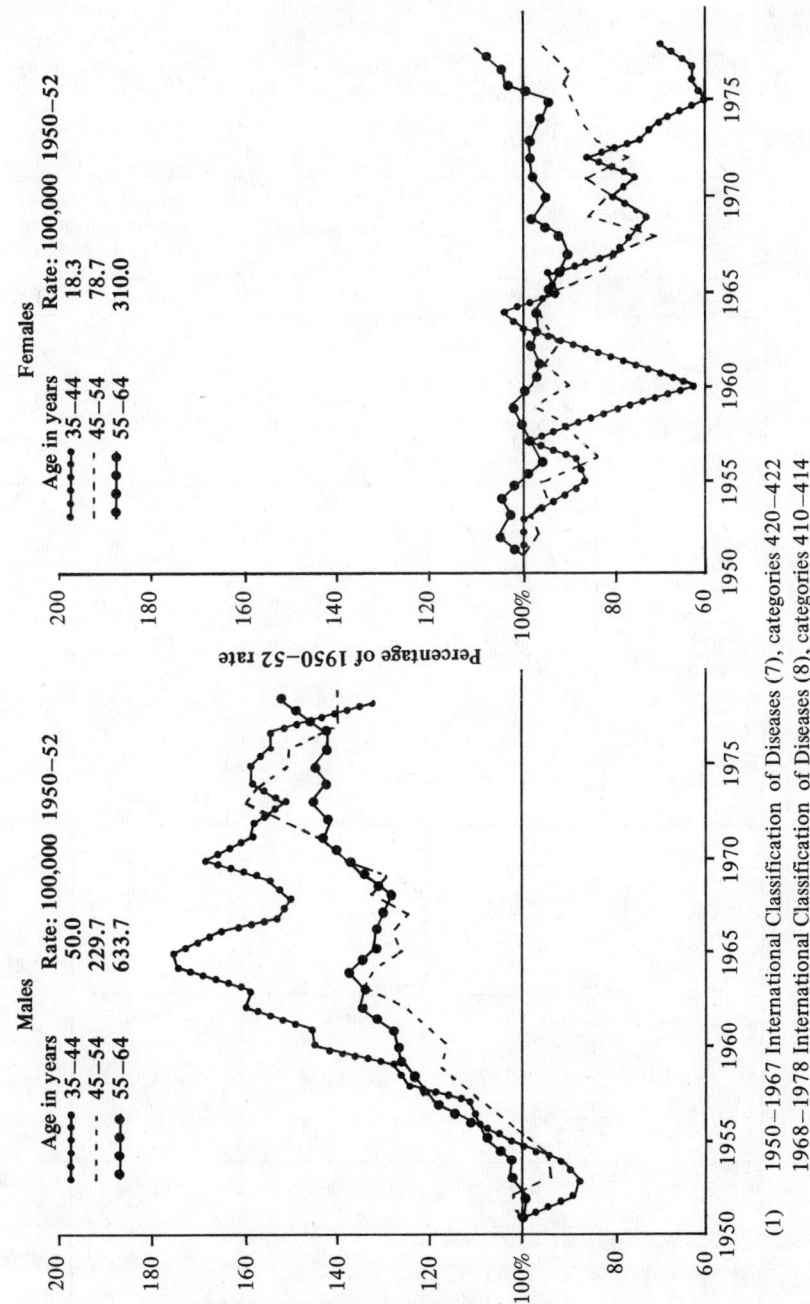

(1) 1950–1967 International Classification of Diseases (7), categories 420–422
    1968–1978 International Classification of Diseases (8), categories 410–414

Fig. 5.   Deaths from coronary heart disease in the United Kingdom by age group and sex, 1978. Numbers and proportion of deaths from all causes.

Number of coronary heart disease deaths		Age group	Coronary heart disease deaths as proportion of all deaths in age group	
Males	Females		Males	Females
222	59	25–34	6%	3%
2,017	360	35–44	29%	8%
9,212	1,799	45–54	41%	13%
22,427	7,099	55–64	39%	21%
37,859	21,187	65–74	34%	28%
105,999	78,820	All ages	32%	24%

Fig. 6. Death rate of males and females from coronary heart disease at ages 15−74 years in 24 countries, 1974−76

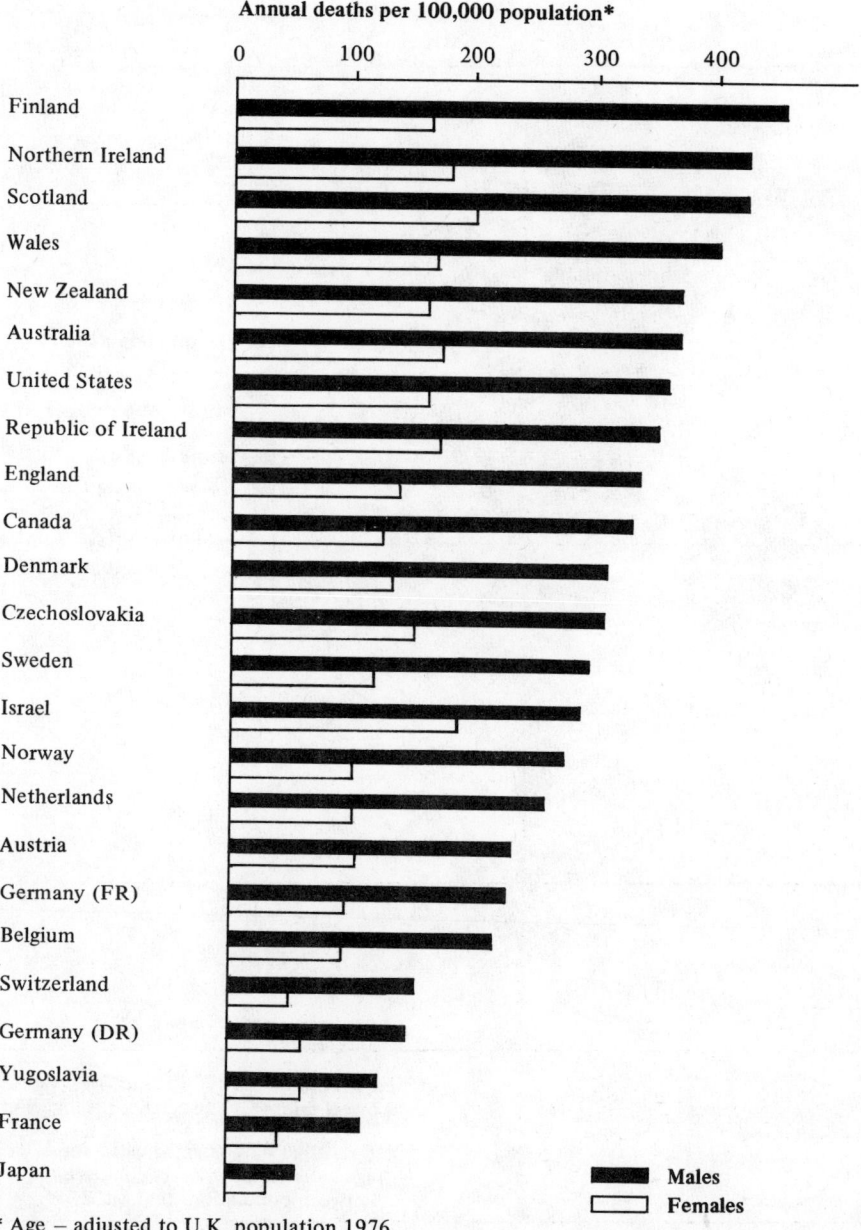

Annual deaths per 100,000 population*

* Age − adjusted to U.K. population 1976.

Fig. 7.   Standardised death rates* from coronary heart disease of males at ages 35 to 64 years, 1969–1973 U.K. regional variations.

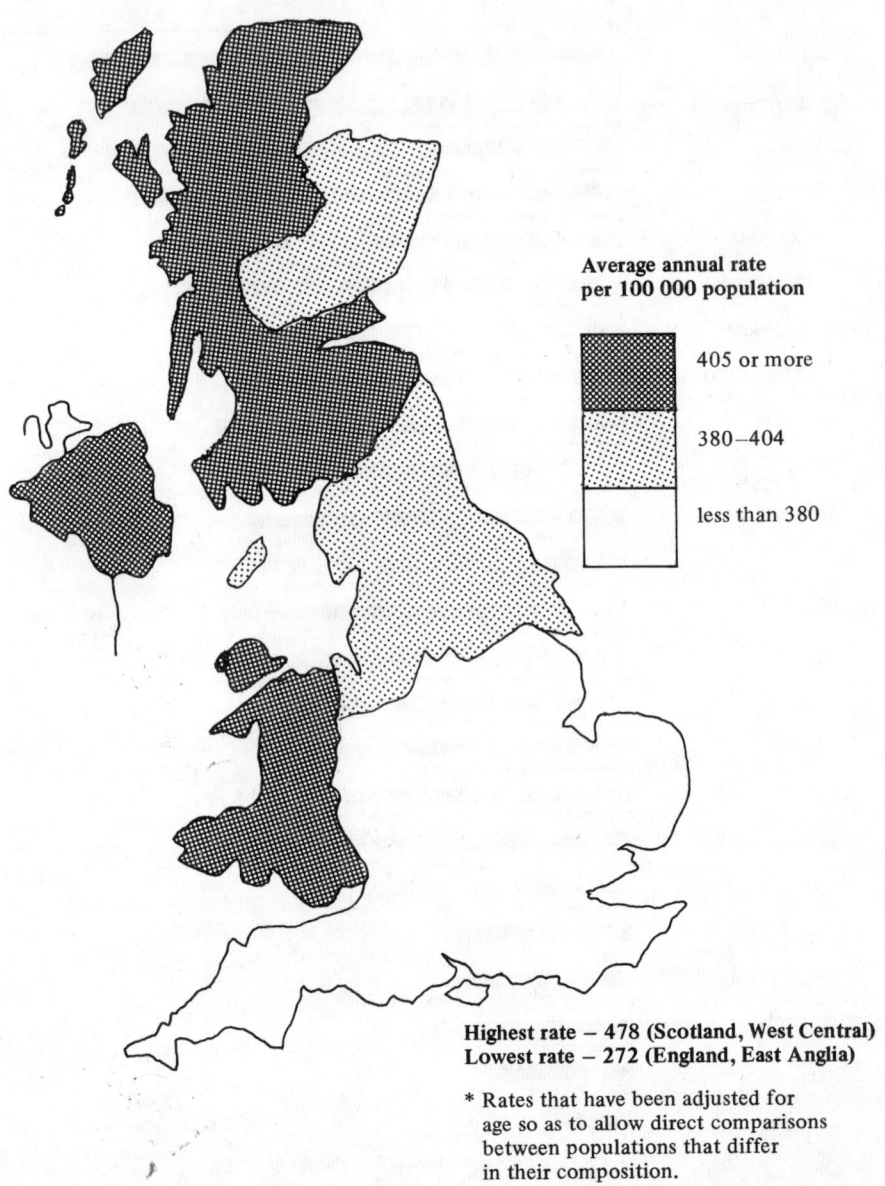

Average annual rate
per 100 000 population

405 or more

380–404

less than 380

Highest rate – 478 (Scotland, West Central)
Lowest rate – 272 (England, East Anglia)

* Rates that have been adjusted for
age so as to allow direct comparisons
between populations that differ
in their composition.

CHAPTER IV Factors that increase the risk

Despite the enormous amount of research over the past 30 years or so, no one knows the cause of coronary heart disease. The views of experts, be it on diet, exercise, heredity, smoking, stress or whatever, inevitably make headlines. Small wonder if the ordinary citizen is often confused by the multiplicity of opinions.

Risk factors and causes

A risk factor is any characteristic of an individual that has been observed by past experience to increase the risk of that person developing a disease or having an accident or, in general, of having something specified happen to him or her. For that person the risk, whatever its nature, is higher than it is for the person who does not possess that particular characteristic. As we have already seen, men are more liable than women to develop coronary heart disease. We could say therefore that being male is a risk factor for this disease. Similarly, we know that older people are more liable than younger people to heart attacks. Age is, therefore, also a risk factor. But not all men develop coronary heart disease and not all women escape; some young men get the disease while others live to an advanced age and may get knocked down by a bus. It follows that these characteristics, sex and age, cannot be fully responsible for coronary heart disease. It is in this sense that we must admit that no one knows what *the* cause of coronary heart disease really is.

Indeed, it is almost certain that there is no one single cause but a multiplicity of causal factors which when present in various degrees and combinations produce the disease. This complexity is not a reason for giving up. From the point of view of prevention, it is valuable to know what the risk factors are, because the removal of some of these factors may reduce the risk of the disease developing.

Research into heart disease

We cannot do much about such risk factors as our sex and age or, insofar as heredity may contribute to the incidence of the disease, about the genes which determine our inherited characteristics. But there are other risk factors which we might be able to influence. In order to find ways in which risk factors can be recognised and to find out whether modification or removal of these risk factors really does reduce the risk of coronary heart disease, scientists have proceeded in 3 stages.

The first stage involves making comparisons between patients who already have the disease and a second group, called the 'control' group (matched as carefully as possible for age and sex), who are free of it. The investigators then try and establish any characteristics, for example a physical characteristic such as blood pressure, or a way of life, by which the 2 groups differ. Such a study, because it looks at factors that may have already had their effect, is called a *retrospective study*.

The second stage, after deciding which characteristics are worth investigating further, is to enrol a group of individuals, usually volunteers, and follow them up for several years, first carefully noting for each individual the presence or absence of characteristics being investigated. We can then relate the fate of the individual—that is, whether he did not develop the disease—to his characteristics on enrolment. For example, we might record the blood pressure of each volunteer on entry to the study and see whether, in the outcome, those with the high blood pressure fared worse than those whose blood pressure was normal or low. Such a study is, for obvious reasons, called a *prospective study*. At the end of such a study one might have, for example, a high degree of suspicion concerning blood pressure. If so, high blood pressure has now become a *risk factor*. In other words, those with high blood pressure have a greater *chance*—a higher risk—of developing the disease we are interested in. We have not yet *proved* that this risk factor is also a cause. It may be entirely co-incidental. For that we must move on to the third phase.

The third stage, then, is to try and discover whether removing or modifying the risk factor will help to prevent the disease. If it does so, then the risk factor moves nearer to being a *cause*. Such an experiment is a special sort of prospective study, called an *intervention study*. A group of volunteers is enrolled and divided randomly into two groups. People in one group undergo some procedure (for instance medication or health education) to try and remove or lessen some of their risk factors. They are then compared with people in the other group who did not undergo this procedure. Ideally this kind of study should be able to tell us, firstly, whether the procedure adopted has been successful in modifying risk factors and, secondly, how effective that modification has been in preventing the disease from developing. Thus, in the example given, the experimental group might be given a drug to reduce the blood pressure. We should then want to know, firstly, whether the drug is successful in doing just that and, secondly, and of greater importance, whether reducing the blood pressure reduces the incidence of the disease.

What do the studies show?

It must be admitted that results to date have not been particularly conclusive as far as coronary heart disease is concerned. Indeed, some experts have expressed doubts as to whether we shall ever attain scientific certainty about even the best-recognised risk factors for this disease. Even accepting this pessimistic view does not mean that we cannot take preventive action. After all, we are accustomed, though we may not always recognise it, to take our decisions on the basis of what we think is likely to happen rather than on what we are sure will happen.

There are no tests that would have allowed us to predict even a few hours in advance with any certainty that the late J B Smith, whose death we read about at the beginning of this booklet, was about to have that fatal heart attack last February. Knowing certain facts about him would have enabled us, however, to assess the probability that he was going to have a heart attack in the foreseeable future. At least we knew that J B Smith was a male aged 41, and that the present UK yearly coronary death rate of males between 40 and 44 years is about one per 1000. There was therefore a thousand to one chance against any man in that age range, J B Smith included, dying from a coronary within the next 12 months.

However he may have been at greater risk and if we knew more about J B Smith we might be able to sharpen up our prediction about him. We started with the group defined as 'males aged 40−44 years in England and Wales' and that by itself was not a very useful predictor. The group have a variety of characteristics; some are rich, others are poor; some are fat, others thin; some drink, others do not; some have blue eyes, others brown; and so on. We could sub-divide into smaller and smaller groups. If we knew enough about J B Smith to assign him to a particular sub-group and we knew the probability of a heart attack for the members generally of that sub-group, we could assess his risk of a heart attack better than if all we knew was his age and where he lived.

Scientific studies have indicated the characteristics that appear to matter in defining sub-groups and refining our estimates of the chances of coronary heart disease. As it happens, eye colour is not one of them but the list is varied and the characteristics implicated in one or more studies are set out in Table 1. Not all the experts agree on all the factors and many studies have been confined to examine one, or at most 2 or 3 at a time. No study has ever been reported that took all the factors into account and it is unlikely that any ever will. Almost all the reported studies agree that the first 3 factors in Table 1, namely, cigarette smoking, blood pressure and the level of cholesterol in the blood (see Chapter VII), are important, and furthermore that each acts independently and exerts its effect no matter what the level of the other factors may be. How much importance one should attach to the risk factors other than the 3 main ones, is a matter of dispute, although it is increasingly accepted that they are of secondary effect.

Nevertheless, the studies do help to sort out the very considerable complexities and allow us to recognise the existence of risk factors and to assess their relative importance. In the chapters that follow, the evidence for the existence of the main risk factors for coronary heart disease is examined so that the reader can decide for himself whether he should himself act upon it in the hope of avoiding, or at least of postponing, a coronary heart attack. And, in doing so, he or she will no doubt take into account not only the strength of the evidence about any particular risk factor but also the importance of what is at stake: it may be a matter of life or death.

Table 1 Risk factors for coronary heart disease

Note: In most cases of coronary heart disease it is likely that more than one factor is present. Only the first three characteristics given below have been shown to operate as risk factors independently of others. A combination of factors is likely to increase the risk.

	Characteristic	Effect on the risk of coronary heart disease
Principal risk factors	Smoking (cigarettes)	The greater the amount smoked currently, the greater the risk
	Blood pressure	The higher the pressure the greater the risk
	Blood cholesterol	The greater the concentration the greater the risk
	Diabetes	People with diabetes have a higher risk
	Family history	The longer parents live, the less the risk for their children
	Obesity	Being overweight *may* increase the risk (unproven)
	Stress	Stress *may* increase the risk (unproven)
	Personality	Some types *may* be more prone than others (unproven)
	Physical activity	The less exercise customarily taken, the greater *may* be the risk (unproven)
	Hardness of tap water	The softer the tap water the greater *may* be the risk (unproven)

CHAPTER V Smoking

Cigarette smoking is a powerful and independent risk factor for coronary heart disease, particularly at younger ages. This is the verdict of every propective investigation that has taken smoking into account, and most of them have done so. Because the reference is to cigarette smoking it should not be assumed that other forms of smoking are entirely free from risk so far as the disease is concerned. Pipe smokers may be at slightly higher risk than non-smokers. The risks attached to smoking cigars are not so easy to judge, partly because there have been comparatively few studies of cigar smokers. Cigarillos have become popular too recently for there to be any evidence one way or another. There is however a strong suggestion that what matters is not the form in which the tobacco is used but the amount of smoke inhaled.

How smoking affects the heart

People can readily visualise how smoking can affect the lungs and give rise to smoker's cough, bronchitis, and lung cancer. It is obvious that the smoke itself is bound to get into direct contact with the tissues of the lung, particularly if the smoker inhales. It is not so obvious why smoking should affect the heart, acting at a distance as it were. The answer may lie in the complex nature of tobacco smoke. As many as 2000 different chemical substances can be detected by analysis in tobacco smoke, with minute solid particles and tiny oily droplets (tar) suspended in a complex mixture of gases produced from the burning material. Some of these chemicals are arrested in the lung but others pass through into the bloodstream and are carried along to the heart, as well as to other organs, like the brain. At least two of these substances—and there may well be several others—are known to have direct effects on the heart—nicotine and carbon monoxide.

Nicotine acts in some respects like an injection of adrenalin; the pulse rate quickens, the blood pressure goes up, and the heart muscle demands more oxygen. This in turn calls for an increased flow down the coronary arteries. Indeed, the coronary arteries can actually expand under the influence of nicotine to allow for this increased flow, *provided they are healthy* and have a normal degree of elasticity. If the arteries are diseased they cannot expand, and the heart muscle does not get enough oxygen until the effect of the nicotine has worn off.

Carbon monoxide gas has the same end result but the lack of oxygen for the heart muscle arises in a different way. The gas links up very firmly, much more firmly than oxygen, with the haemoglobin in the red blood cells and prevents them from picking up and carrying as much oxygen as they would otherwise do. If the amount of carbon monoxide in the blood is allowed to build up to the point where a third or more of the haemoglobin is affected, death will be rapid. A lesser build-up is not uncommon. Tobacco smoke may contain up to 5 per cent of carbon monoxide and it can lead to a build-up of 10 per cent or even more in the blood of regular smokers, which compares with the 0.5 or 1 per cent usually found in non-smokers. (The carbon monoxide in non-smokers' blood comes from the environment—eg vehicle exhaust fumes and other people's smoking; in some jobs—workers in foundries, drivers of stationary engines, policemen on point duty—non-smokers can build up as much carbon monoxide in the blood as cigarette smokers). As well as reducing the oxygen-carrying capacity of the blood, carbon monoxide has another potentially harmful effect on the heart; it impedes the release of oxygen at the point of need. Not only is less oxygen than usual transported, but this reduced amount is less readily available. Smoking also appears to disturb the nervous mechanism which helps to control the heart beat. The effect of this disturbance can range from the relatively innocuous palpitations sometimes experienced by people smoking more than they are used to, to the extreme of sudden death.

Smoking and the increased risk of heart disease
When the effect of smoking on health first started to attract attention in the 1940s the focus was almost exclusively on lung diseases, especially lung cancer. As the evidence accumulated it became obvious that smoking affected the heart in at least as many cases as it affected the lungs. As early as 1951 a relationship was shown between smoking and coronary heart disease, and this connection has been repeatedly confirmed since then.

The pooled results of five American studies have been used to prepare Figure 8 which shows how in each smoking category the incidence of coronary heart disease increases with age, and how at each age the incidence is dependent on smoking category, being at all points lowest among non-smokers and highest among those who smoked the most. These rates, which are based on the follow-up for an average of eight and a half years of 8500 men, all initially free of signs of heart disease, show that of every three men who at the age of 40 were heavy smokers one will have had a major heart

Fig. 8. Out of every 1,000 men aged 40 to 60 years the number who will develop coronary heart disease[1] within the next five years, by smoking category (based on Pooling Project Research Group Report, 1978).

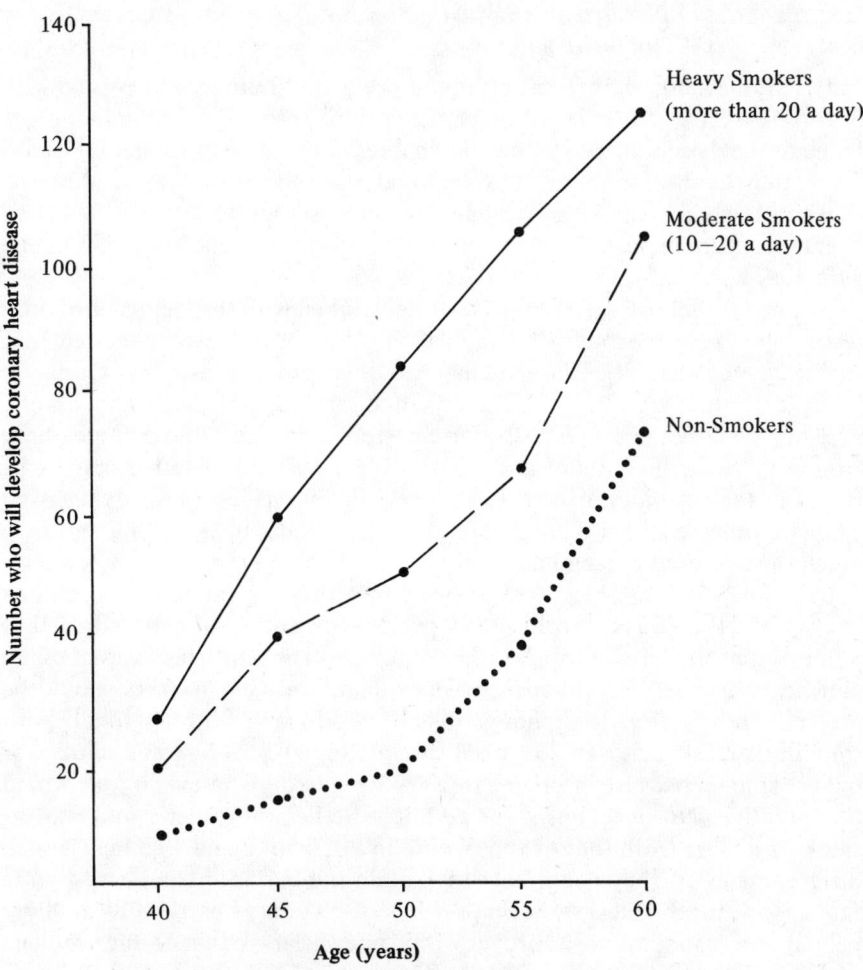

[1] Coronary heart disease = acute heart attack (myocardial infarction) or sudden death

attack (probably fatal) before he reaches 65 whilst six out of seven non-smokers will have reached that age without a heart attack.

Many studies have now shown that the risk of coronary heart disease for smokers, compared with the risk for non-smokers,—

increases with the amount smoked;

is detectable even among those smoking on average as few as 5 – 10 a day;

may be twenty times as great for really heavy smokers (two packets a day);

is reduced to not much more than the risk for lifelong non-smokers within a few years of giving up smoking.

The studies also show that, although the actual numbers of people with heart disease are greater in the older age groups, the younger a smoker is the higher is the risk compared to the non-smoker of the same age: it is very rare to encounter the disease in non-smokers under 40. From the age of about 60 onwards the relative risk for non-smokers increases until by the age of 65 and over there is not much difference between someone who smokes and someone who does not.

Evidently, therefore, smoking is strongly linked with the incidence of, and death rate from, coronary heart disease, and it has been suggested that smoking may actually cause damage to the coronary arteries. Certainly damage to the arteries is more common among smokers than among non-smokers. Some large post-mortem studies in the United States have established that the amount and extent of disease patches (atheroma) to be found in the coronary arteries of people killed in accidents, or dying from causes unrelated to smoking is directly proportional to how long and how much the deceased person had smoked.

But some studies suggest that smokers may differ from non-smokers in a variety of other ways, in physique, personality and social characteristics. Some of these differences might account for the connection between smoking and heart disease—in which case the explanation why smokers should be affected more often than non-smokers could have nothing to do with smoking itself. If that were so it would not matter whether a person smoked or did not smoke, because in either case the other factor, whatever it was, would be operative. No-one knows for certain whether the genetic make-up of smokers differs from that of those who do not smoke and whether, if such differences exist, they could help to explain the variations in heart disease rates. However the facts show that the risk of coronary heart disease in those people who stop smoking improves within a few years to that of non-smokers and their genetic make-up remains the same. That people vary in their susceptibility to the effects of tobacco is pretty obvious—we have all heard of that legendary figure, the man who has been smoking 40 a day all his life and is none the worse for it though he is pushing 90! The relative risk for smokers is greatest at younger ages and one explanation why that should be is that those most suspectible to the harmful effects of tobacco are the ones to be picked off first.

Nevertheless, it can be said as a result of several studies carried out in Britain, Israel and the United States that, as a risk factor, smoking is independent of the other two main factors, blood pressure and blood cholesterol concentrations. Whether a non-smoker's blood pressure is high or normal, he or she has a better chance of escaping the disease than the smoker with the same blood pressure. Similarly, whether the cholesterol concentration in the blood is large or small, the smoker is at greater risk than the non-smoker with the same cholesterol concentration.

Trends in smoking

In this and in other industrial countries cigarette smoking became increasingly popular in the years from World War I onwards, and by the end of World War II two out of three adult males in Britain were cigarette smokers. During the 1960s and 1970s the proportion of adult men who were regular smokers tended to decline and by 1980 the percentage was down to 42 per cent. Among women the proportion remained fairly steady around the 40–45 per cent mark from the late 1950s to 1972, and this was followed by a very slow decline to 1980 when it was 37 per cent. Although about a third of 16–19 year olds smoke cigarettes, it is encouraging that an increasing proportion of people under 25 have never taken up the habit.

Although the proportion of men who smoke has been falling, and the proportion among women has not changed much, the proportion of smokers of both sexes who smoke heavily has increased markedly over the past 20 years. In the last 25 years the average consumption by each cigarette smoker has gone up by about 20 per cent for men and by about 70 per cent for women.

These changes have not affected all social classes to the same extent. Over the past 15 years the drop in proportion of smokers has been very much more marked among professional people of both sexes and the message has not yet got across to the rest of the population to anything like the same degree.

By and large these trends fit in well enough with some of the facts about coronary heart disease which have been noted. Thus, the rising frequency of the disease over the past half century has followed the increase in popularity of the cigarette and the shift away from pipe smoking. Again the recent downward trend in the death rate among younger men, not seen to the same extent among women (Figure 4), would correspond with the changes in smoking habits. The most striking change in death rates from the disease is that recorded for doctors, who in 1931 had a rate several times that of men in general; by 1971 their rate was below that of all men. By contrast the death rate for semi-skilled workers as a group increased steadily over the same span of four decades. It has been plausibly suggested that changes in society—particularly economic changes—over the period have enabled the semi-skilled worker increasingly to adopt the harmful habit of smoking that doctors used to indulge in but have tended more and more to avoid.

The benefits of stopping smoking

There are many good reasons why a smoker should give up smoking but the question we are concerned with here is whether, if he does so, his chances of avoiding a coronary would improve. The short answer is that they would. A now classic study of British doctors, who were followed up for 25 years, showed that those who gave up smoking cigarettes before the age of 55 could expect after 5 years to reduce their risk of fatal coronary heart disease to less than half what it would have been. (The time of 5 years had to be allowed so as to avoid counting those who had given up smoking for reasons of existing ill-health). After the age of 55 ceasing to smoke had not such a marked effect in reducing the risk, even though it was still detectable. American studies have shown similar results. There is therefore an advantage in giving up smoking cigarettes even for those who have smoked for many years; and the younger the habit is dropped the better. Best of all, of course, is not to start in the first place. The dangers for women of smoking are discussed in more detail in Chapter IX.

For the smoker who finds it so hard to give up that he cannot help but continue, a practical question is whether the risk to health can be reduced. For some years now the Department of Health has published periodically a list giving the tar and nicotine yield of different cigarette brands on the market. No single smoke component has been causally linked with coronary heart disease, but nicotine and carbon monoxide have long been suspected. Nevertheless the evidence on individual smoke components is controversial. From what has been said earlier, there are grounds for thinking that the low nicotine brands may have a somewhat lesser effect on the heart beat rate. Another component of smoke which may affect the heart—carbon monoxide—is not held back, as tar is to some extent, by an ordinary filter. The manner of smoking, the number and frequency of puffs, could well determine the level of carbon monoxide in the inhaled smoke to a greater extent than the tobacco mixture. While it is likely that a 'ventilated' filter ensures that less carbon monoxide is delivered, it would require a large long-term study to show what value, if any, this would have so far as coronary heart disease goes. Recent data from studies in the United States suggests that there is no evidence that filters confer any protection from coronary heart disease.

As far as low tar products are concerned, these only came into commercial use in recent years and there is not yet enough evidence on the risks of coronary heart disease associated with them. In the meantime it cannot be assumed that switching to low tar cigarettes removes all risk of the disease. The safest course is to quit.

CHAPTER VI Blood pressure

Every prospective study to date agrees that the level of a person's blood pressure (the pressure maintained within the arteries by the action of the heart pumping the blood) will give a good indication of his or her risk of developing coronary heart disease. As we grow older our blood pressure tends to rise but, even allowing for this age-effect, the chances of suffering a heart attack increase steadily with every increase in blood pressure. A number of studies throughout the world have shown that people whose blood pressure is in the top 20 per cent of the range have a risk of coronary heart disease about twice that of people with a pressure in the bottom 20 per cent. A high blood pressure (hypertension) seems to be a stronger risk factor at older ages, and to be just as important for women as for men. The studies also indicate that high blood pressure is a risk factor independent of the other factors such as cigarette smoking and a high blood cholesterol concentration. Indeed, some experts consider that it is second only to smoking as a risk factor.

How exactly a high blood pressure leads to heart disease is a matter of some dispute. According to one explanation the effect is purely mechanical; the linings of the arteries are damaged as the result of the constant excessive hammering they receive when the blood pressure is higher than it should be. At post-mortem of people with high blood pressure, patches of disease (atheroma) are to be found at just those points—bends and kinks in the blood vessels—where maximum turbulence would occur in the blood stream.

The cause of high blood pressure is also in dispute and there may be a number of causes—some preventable, others not. But blood pressure can be reduced by reduction of weight in the obese and by limiting the amount of salt in the diet (see Chapter VII). From the records of insurance companies it has long been known that people with high blood pressure have on average a lower life expectancy than their contemporaries with normal blood pressure. Depending on just how high the blood pressure is the life expectancy of a 35 year old may be reduced by 40 per cent. This is not only due to coronary heart disease but also to other consequences of high blood pressure, such as strokes and kidney failure.

Nowadays there are effective drugs for lowering the blood pressure; and treating high blood pressure will certainly reduce the frequency of these other conditions. There is also some evidence that such treatment can help specifically to prevent coronary heart disease. Control of high blood pressure can therefore be an important part of disease prevention. Whether the undoubted benefits of treating very high blood pressure apply also to the treatment of moderately raised blood pressure is as yet unknown and research is being conducted to find out. Nevertheless it is wise to have blood pressure checks from time to time.

Treatment of moderately raised blood pressure by drugs may not be necessary and much can be achieved by modifying habits that are likely to predispose to raised blood pressure. Excessive alcohol intake not only leads to weight increase but it has on its own been associated with high blood pressure so it is important to avoid heavy drinking. A reduction in the amount of salt added to food and avoiding an excessive increase in body weight are also reasonable steps to take to help maintain normal blood pressure.

CHAPTER VII Eating and the heart

In broad terms, people are made up of the food and drink they consume. This applies to the heart muscle and coronary arteries as well as to other parts of the body. The relationship between diet and coronary heart disease still generates argument and controversy. Over the years, many expert committees, national and international, have offered advice on what should be done regarding diet, both by Governments and individuals, in order to reduce the toll of the disease. On the whole there is a fair measure of agreement, but this is by no means total, and there always seem to be some experts who will draw a different conclusion from the same set of facts. It is small wonder that the layman is sometimes left in a state of confusion.

It may help to clarify the issues by considering the main factors looked at by these expert groups:

a. total food energy;
b. fats, including saturated and polyunsaturated fatty acids, and cholesterol;
c. sugar;
d. dietary fibre;
e. salt;
f. alcohol;
g. water.

Total food energy

For every individual there is thought to be an 'ideal' weight. This depends on the person's age, body build (or 'frame'), height and sex. A table of ideal weights, based on the records kept by American insurance companies of the measurements of American people who lived the longest, is given at Table 2. By definition, people whose weight differed from the ideal, in either direction, must have been less likely to live so long. In particular, the more overweight they were, the more likely they were to die prematurely. This is why experts recommend that everyone should strive to achieve and keep to the weight considered to be ideal for his or her height and build.

Table 2   Desirable weights of adults*

Desirable weight in pounds and *Kilogrammes* (in indoor clothing), ages 25 and over

Height (in shoes)		Small frame		Medium frame		Large frame	
ft in	*cm*	lb	*kg*	lb	*kg*	lb	*kg*
			MEN				
5 2	*157.5*	112–120	*50.8–54.4*	118–129	*53.5–58.5*	126–141	*57.2–64*
5 3	*160*	115–123	*52.2–55.8*	121–133	*54.9–60.3*	129–144	*58.5–65.3*
5 4	*162.6*	118–126	*53.5–57.2*	124–136	*56.2–64.7*	132–148	*59.9–67.1*
5 5	*165.1*	121–129	*54.9–58.5*	127–139	*57.6–63*	135–152	*61.2–68.9*
5 6	*167.6*	124–133	*56.2–60.3*	130–143	*59 –64.9*	138–156	*62.6–70.8*
5 7	*170.2*	128–137	*58.1–62.1*	134–147	*60.8–66.7*	142–161	*64.4–73*
5 8	*172.7*	132–141	*59.9–64*	138–152	*62.6–68.9*	147–166	*66.7–75.3*
5 9	*175.3*	136–145	*61.7–65.8*	142–156	*64.4–70.8*	151–170	*68.5–77.1*
5 10	*177.8*	140–150	*63.5–68*	146–160	*66.2–72.6*	155–174	*70.3–78.9*
5 11	*180.3*	144–154	*65.3–69.9*	150–165	*68 –74.8*	159–179	*72.1–81.2*
6 0	*182.9*	148–158	*67.1–71.7*	154–170	*69.9–77.1*	164–184	*74.4–83.5*
6 1	*185.4*	152–162	*68.9–73.5*	158–175	*71.7–79.4*	168–189	*76.2–85.7*
6 2	*188*	156–167	*70.8–75.7*	162–180	*73.5–81.6*	173–194	*78.5–88*
6 3	*190.5*	160–171	*72.6–77.6*	167–185	*75.7–83.5*	178–199	*80.7–90.3*
6 4	*193*	164–175	*74.4–79.4*	172–190	*78.1–86.2*	182–204	*82.7–92.5*
			WOMEN				
4 10	*147.3*	92– 98	*41.7–44.5*	96–107	*43.5–48.5*	104–119	*47.2–54*
4 11	*149.9*	94–101	*42.6–45.8*	98–110	*44.5–49.9*	106–122	*48.1–55.3*
5 0	*152.4*	96–104	*43.5–47.2*	101–113	*45.8–51.3*	109–125	*49.4–56.7*
5 1	*154.9*	99–107	*44.9–48.5*	104–116	*47.2–52.6*	112–128	*50.8–58.1*
5 2	*157.5*	102–110	*46.3–49.9*	107–119	*48.5–54*	115–131	*52.2–59.4*
5 3	*160*	105–113	*47.6–51.3*	110–122	*49.9–55.3*	118–134	*53.5–60.8*
5 4	*162.6*	108–116	*49 –52.6*	113–126	*51.3–57.2*	121–138	*54.9–62.6*
5 5	*165.1*	111–119	*50.3–54*	116–130	*52.7–59*	125–142	*56.8–64.4*
5 6	*167.6*	114–123	*51.7–55.8*	120–135	*54.4–61.2*	129–146	*58.5–66.2*
5 7	*170.2*	118–127	*53.5–57.6*	124–139	*56.2–63*	133–150	*60.3–68*
5 8	*172.7*	122–131	*55.3–59.4*	128–143	*58.1–64.9*	137–154	*62.1–69.9*
5 9	*175.3*	126–135	*57.2–61.2*	132–147	*59.9–66.7*	141–158	*64 –71.7*
5 10	*177.8*	130–140	*59 –63.5*	136–151	*61.7–68.5*	145–163	*65.8–73.9*
5 11	*180.3*	134–144	*60.8–65.3*	140–155	*63.5–70.3*	149–168	*67.6–76.2*
6 0	*182.9*	138–148	*62.6–67.1*	144–159	*65.3–72.1*	153–173	*69.4–78.5*

* Weights of insured persons in the United States associated with lowest mortality.

From Society of Actuaries, 1959. Average weights and heights. In Build and Blood Pressure Study, Volume I, compiled by the Society of Actuaries p.16 Chicago, Society of Actuaries. Reproduced from Eating for Health (HMSO 1978) p.59.

Although obese people, especially men in early middle life, are at greater risk of many diseases, including coronary heart disease, none of the major studies has shown that obesity *by itself* is an important risk factor, or a reliable predictor of coronary heart disease. But obese people often possess other relevant characteristics, such as a raised blood pressure or a tendency to diabetes. They may take little physical exercise. It is such factors which account for their increased risk. So if the person is free of these other risk factors, no promises of immunity from coronary heart disease can be held out to the obese person who decides to shed weight.

There are, of course, other excellent reasons why one should avoid being overweight. Most people who have lost their superfluous weight will testify that they gained in more than one way. The basic formula is simple enough for most people: if energy in-take equals energy expenditure, body weight stays constant: if in-take exceeds expenditure, weight goes up; while if in-take is less than expenditure, weight is lost. It is the balance of energy in-take and expenditure that matters.* The booklet *Eating for Health* gives practical advice for the overweight person to help achieve the ideal weight.

Fats and cholesterol

In the United Kingdom we eat a lot of fat. It provides about 38% of total food energy. Countries which eat a Western-type diet, rich in fat, are also those in which the death rate from coronary heart disease is high. The statistical evidence for some association between a diet rich in fat and the death rate from the disease fits in with experimental evidence: when monkeys were fed a typical Western high-fat diet, they developed a disease of the arteries like, although not identical to, coronary heart disease in humans.

The fats that we eat (including edible oils) come from three sources: plants, land animals and marine animals. In chemical terms, all the fats and oils are compounds of fatty acids and they may be classified according to whether they contain a predominance of saturated or polyunsaturated fatty acids. Many animal fats, like butter, suet and beef dripping are rich in saturated fatty acids but low in polyunsaturated acids. Some, like pork and poultry, contain somewhat less of saturated fatty acids and a little more polyunsaturated acids. Fish oils, on the other hand, are moderate to rich in polyunsaturated fatty acids. Some vegetable oils, such as coconut oil, contain almost entirely saturated fatty acids. And some such as corn oil, sunflower oil, soya bean oil and cottonseed oil are rich in polyunsaturated fatty acids.

Dietary fat is transported in the blood stream after ingestion, stored in fatty tissues, and is released and burnt as energy when needed. Cholesterol is

---

* See Table 3, Chapter 8, for a comparison of some food intakes and physical activities which are roughly equivalent in energy value.

one part of this fat. Cholesterol is a component of cell membranes and is the basic substance from which the body is able to build certain hormones. Obviously, therefore, the body must have a pool of cholesterol constantly available.

The importance of the concentration of cholesterol in the blood as a risk factor for coronary heart disease has already been mentioned (page 30). It has long been known that communities with a low death rate from heart attacks are those in which the concentration of cholesterol in the blood is on average lower than that found in people from North America and Western Europe. The hypothesis has been put forward, though not proved, that a diet rich in fat, particularly in saturated fatty acids, may lead to an increase in the concentration of cholesterol in the blood and to the accumulation of cholesterol in the walls of arteries where the lining has been damaged. These diseased patches in the coronary arteries may be the root trouble in coronary heart disease, because blood clots develop easily on these areas.

Most of the cholesterol in the blood is manufactured by the body itself and is not derived from the diet at all but experiments have shown that raised blood cholesterol can be reduced by one of several different dietary changes. An overweight person can reduce his blood cholesterol by decreasing his total food intake so that he is no longer overweight. Blood cholesterol can also be reduced by a reduction of total dietary fat, especially by a reduction of saturated fatty acids from both animal and vegetable sources, but also by substituting certain vegetable oils containing mainly polyunsaturated fatty acids for some animal and vegetable fats containing chiefly saturated fatty acids. Reducing the saturated fatty acids in the diet decreases blood cholesterol more effectively than adding polyunsaturated fatty acids.

Much of the cholesterol in the United Kingdom diet is derived from eggs. But few nutritionists in this country consider that blood cholesterol would be appreciably altered by any change in the number of eggs which are eaten. This is, at present, an average of 4 to 5 per person per week (one of the eggs being contained in cakes and pastry). Other sources are butter, liver and meat. Small changes in dietary cholesterol have little effect on the concentration of blood cholesterol, although extremes of intake, such as 10–12 eggs a day, or none at all, may have a temporary effect.

One dietary change which has been suggested in the hope of reducing the occurrence of heart attacks is the partial substitution of polyunsaturated fatty acids for. saturated fatty acids. In 1974 the Department of Health and Social Security published a report *Diet and Coronary Heart Disease,* prepared by an advisory panel to the Committee on Medical Aspects of Food Policy. The majority of panel members recommended that the amount of fat in the UK diet (especially saturated fat, from both animal and plant sources) should be reduced. But the panel was unanimous 'in remaining unconvinced by the available evidence that the incidence of coronary heart disease in the United Kingdom, or the death rate from it, would be reduced in consequence of a rise in the ratio of polyunsaturated to saturated fatty acids in the national diet'. The panel also concluded that there was no single factor in the diet which was predominant in making people more susceptible to the disease. Any claim, in the context of the United Kingdom diet, that eating, or not eating, a particular food would lower the risk of an individual getting a coronary heart attack, would be unjustified.

In 1976, a working party of the Royal College of Physicians and the British Cardiac Society published a report *The Prevention of Coronary Heart Disease* which discussed diet as one of the risk factors. This report also recommended that the total amount of fat, and especially of saturated fat, in the diet should be reduced. However the working party also considered that, given present tastes in diet, many people might not find a reduction in saturated fat (sufficient to produce a significant fall in blood cholesterol) acceptable unless they put some polyunsaturated fat in their diet instead. The report therefore recommended that people at risk of coronary heart disease should replace some foods rich in saturated fatty acids with those rich in polyunsaturated fatty acids.

In 1977 the Committee on Medical Aspects of Food Policy reconsidered and endorsed its 1974 recommendations. A review of diet and cardiovascular disease is to be undertaken shortly by an advisory panel to the Committee.

To summarise what can be said about fats and heart disease, research findings have not yet provided the complete answer, but the balance of opinion is that it would be wise to reduce the amount of fat, especially fats rich in saturated fatty acids, in the diet. Other changes which might be made in the diet to replace food energy from fat with energy from foods rich in dietary fibre (for example wholemeal bread) could also be beneficial to health.

Sugar
Not one of the expert committees has specifically recommended cutting down on the amount of sugar in the diet as a direct way of preventing coronary heart disease. However, several agree on two relevant points. Firstly, there are other good reasons for avoiding excessive sugar in the diet, such as preventing weight problems and dental decay (especially important in childhood). Secondly, the calories lost by reducing the amount of fat in the diet should be obtained not from refined carbohydrates like sugar, but by increasing the amount of complex, unrefined carbohydrate foods eaten which contain a higher proportion of dietary fibre, such as wholewheat breakfast cereal,

porridge, rice, potatoes and bread (preferably brown or wholemeal) etc. (though some of these may contain some added sugar).

Dietary Fibre

Dietary fibre is the name commonly given to the unabsorbed residue in the fruits, vegetables and cereals we eat. This residue used to be regarded as nutritionally unimportant, until it was realised that in those countries, especially Africa, where the diet traditionally contained a lot of fibre, the so-called 'diseases of civilisation' appeared to be less common. Nutritionists then displayed a special interest in dietary fibre and its possible relationship to human health.

The precise effect of fibre on coronary heart disease is at present unknown. One recent study suggested that of middle-aged men those who usually ate relatively little fibre were more prone to the disease than those who consumed more.

It is true that if less fat and sugar are eaten, the loss of food energy can be made good by eating more cereal food like bread, and fresh fruit and vegetables. But whatever the benefits that might result from eating more fibre in preventing constipation, piles and some bowel diseases, no one could promise that such a dietary change alone would necessarily reduce the risk of illness or death from coronary heart disease. However, a modification of the diet along the lines suggested in this chapter will make an important contribution to the overall reduction of risk.

Salt

One of the three main risk factors for coronary heart disease is high blood pressure. Experiments have shown that excessive salt in the diet of a species of young rats for even a short time can cause high blood pressure in the animals when adult. A diet low in salt not only reinforces the effect of anti-hypertensive drugs for people with high blood pressure but by itself can be an effective treatment. It is also known that high blood pressure is uncommon among people such as the Eskimos of Alaska, and inhabitants of one of the Japanese islands, who do not customarily add salt to their food; whereas other people in Japan and others who live in areas where salt intake is high have a higher blood pressure. Because too much salt may, therefore, raise the blood pressure, and high blood pressure is a danger signal for coronary heart disease, several expert groups have recommended a restriction in salt intake as a further possible way of preventing heart attacks. It is probable that the average person's consumption of common salt is many times as much as the body needs. There would be no risk of a deficiency, therefore, if we were to reduce considerably the amount of salt we add to our food and the consumption of foods with a high salt content such as savoury snacks and by doing so we may be helping to reduce the risk of heart disease. An exception must be made for those engaged in heavy work in humid conditions; they may lose as much as five to seven grams of salt in sweating, and that has to be made good.

Alcohol

There is a well recognised although comparatively rare form of heart disease which afflicts some heavy drinkers. Otherwise there is only scanty and contradictory evidence of a link between alcohol and coronary heart disease. On the whole the experts have been silent on the point. What evidence there is indicates that drinking in moderation does not increase the incidence of coronary heart disease; indeed some studies have indicated a modest reduction in the number of heart attacks amongst moderate drinkers.

There is, however, evidence of an association between heavy drinking and high blood pressure which is, of course, an important risk factor in coronary heart disease. Alcohol also provides a great many calories and heavy drinking can cause difficulties in maintaining ideal weight.

Water

There have been reports in the press from time to time that people who live in soft water areas seem to be slightly more prone to coronary heart disease. It is not known what leads to the slight increase in the disease in such areas. A major study is being conducted in the United Kingdom to try and find out whether something about water really affects coronary heart disease rates.

CHAPTER VIII Don't just sit there!

Most British people today are not much given to strenuous physical effort if it can be avoided. Only 13 per cent walk to work and even fewer go by bicycle. The number of motor cars has, of course, been increasing. The physical demands of even 'heavy' work today are not what they used to be, and the energy demands of most jobs are declining. Nor does the average man expend much energy during his leisure. He spends 20 hours a week (and the average schoolchild spends 24) watching television. The most popular leisure activities are darts and snooker, neither of them highly energetic. Among men under 25 about half engage in no form of outdoor sport whatsoever and 85–90 per cent of all men do not take part in any *active* indoor sport either. The average man walks for 2 miles or more only once every 3 weeks and goes swimming only 3 times a year.

It is natural that scientists should ask whether the fall-off in physical activity might not help to explain the increasing toll of coronary heart disease. There is indeed much evidence that regular exercise seems to provide some protection. The evidence came in the first instance from comparisons of the death rates of men in different occupations, and later from studies of incidence of the disease. In all the comparisons coronary heart disease was more common among the less active than among their more active fellows. Several of the studies covered men in the same industrial group (eg bus drivers and bus conductors) and the comparisons would be relatively free from social class bias.

Because many jobs today are less physically demanding than they used to be some investigators have concentrated on the amount of exercise men take out of working hours. In a study conducted in 1968–70, some 17,000 civil servants of all grades kept a record of their leisure activities. When these records were checked some years later, by which time more than 200 of them had a heart attack, it was found that there had been fewer attacks among the men who had said they habitually engaged in vigorous exercise than the others. Similarly, a recent study of 15,000 men in Ireland found that those engaged in 'heavy' activities in their leisure hours had on average a lower blood pressure and blood cholesterol, were less likely to be overweight and smoked fewer cigarettes than men with moderate leisure activities, while these in turn had a lower score on the risk factors than men with 'minimal' leisure activity.

Comparisons of people with different jobs or leisure activity are difficult to interpret because of the problem of 'self-selection'. That is to say, some of the people in light jobs may have taken those jobs because they already had 'weak' hearts. The apparent connection between taking vigorous exercise and relative freedom from coronary heart disease may have arisen because it was only those people in good 'condition' in the first place who were able to take vigorous exercise.

The capacity of the heart for work can be increased by training so that a standard work-load can be sustained by less effort. One effect of training is to lower the heart rate at rest, thus creating more scope for increased output if required. Another explanation is that the coronary circulation becomes more efficient when the heart is regularly called upon to work at or near its maximum capacity. It is certainly true that really strenuous activity appears to be particularly effective in protecting against *fatal* heart attacks.

In 1977 the European Commission convened a group of experts to consider the role of physical activity in the prevention of coronary heart disease. They found that physical activity was on balance likely to be protective.

Physical exercise may help to prevent a fatal heart attack; but in addition to this, regular exercise brings its own reward and makes one feel more healthy and active.

The energy used up in exercise is expressed in Kilocalories or megajoules,* thus making it possible to compare the expenditure of energy in different activities with the energy intake from the diet. How much energy is used up by the body depends on such things as body weight and the duration and intensity of the activity. Some leisure activities are compared in Table 3. These can only be approximate values for several reasons; for example, the energy used in walking or cycling will vary with the direction and strength of the wind, and that used in swimming will depend on the shape of the body.

Planned courses of exercises show how much exercise is required and how often in order to keep fit. There are several excellent instruction books available, many in paper-back, which describe detailed programmes suitable for men and women of different ages. But here are some guidelines which experts on the subject have put forward—

exercise should be taken regularly and often—at least twice and preferably three times a week;

---

* Where 240 Kilocalories is equal to 1 megajoule

exercise should be strenuous enough to cause breathlessness and sweating. A leisurely four-hour round of golf has less value than forty minutes of hard singles tennis;

plan to work up gradually by stages over a period of 8 to 10 weeks until you reach your optimum level; the aim should be to use up at least 2000 Kilocalories each week on some strenuous physical activity;

you should eventually be able to sustain a short burst of maximum heart output; at that point your heart rate per minute will be approximately equal to 200 less your age; a man of 40 could therefore work up his exercise programme to the pitch when he can tolerate his heart beating at 160 per minute for a short time;

maximum output should not be continued for more than two or three minutes a session, except by highly trained athletes;

exercise involving rhythmic use of the large muscles as in walking and swimming, is preferable to the more static (isometric) muscular effort as in weight lifting or press-ups.

Table 3. Some food intakes and some physical activities which are equivalent in energy value to approximately 1.25 MJ (300 Kcal)*

Energy expenditure 1.25 MJ (300 Kcal)		Energy intake 1.25 MJ (300 Kcal)	
Activity	Time period	Food	Approximate quantity
Golf	2 hours	Sugar	2¾ oz or 18 lumps
Tennis	¼ to 1 hour	Bread	6 slices
Gardening	¼ to 1 hour	Milk	¾ pint
Football	30-40 minutes	Cheese	2½ oz
Competitive swimming	15 minutes	Bacon	3 oz
		Eggs	3 large size
Cross-country running	15 minutes	Potatoes	1 lb
Hill climbing	less than 1 hour	Biscuits	6 digestive biscuits
4 mile walk	1 hour	Gin or Whisky	6 singles
Do-it-yourself house repairs and decorating	3 hours	Beer	2 pints
		Table wine	½ litre (4 glasses)

*1.25 MJ (300 Kcal) is approximately the difference in energy expenditure per day between sedentary and moderately active occupations.

Adapted from "Eating for Health" (HMSO 1978, Table 7.1).

Physical exercise should above all be something to be enjoyed, not suffered. So choose the form of activity that gives the most pleasure, whether it be disco-dancing or climbing mountains. Lots of people prefer some form of group activity such as keep fit classes; others prefer 'jogging'. It is important that exercise should be regular and equally important to avoid sudden bursts of unaccustomed strenuous exercise.

Most people do not need to have a medical examination before starting on a properly graduated exercise programme, that is one that begins gently and increases in vigour in a planned manner. But, of course, if any untoward symptoms develop during the exercise programme these should be checked with a doctor before going on with it. And those who have had any heart trouble in the past, or are under treatment for any reason, should seek their doctor's advice before starting the programme.

CHAPTER IX Women and coronary heart disease

In general, at every age men are more vulnerable than women of the same age. The disparity is very marked up to the age of 50 or so; after that, although the death rate among women starts to increase rapidly with advancing age, the female death rates never quite catch up with those of males (Figure 3). This is true in every country for which information is available (Figure 6) and seems always to have been so as far back as figures have been collected.

The reason for this really quite remarkable difference between the sexes is not known. The main risk factors—high blood pressure, blood cholesterol concentration and cigarette smoking—are risk factors for women just as they are for men. It is true that women, especially at the younger ages, tend on average to have a slightly lower blood pressure than men of the same age, and a somewhat lower blood cholesterol, and that slightly fewer women than men smoke cigarettes. However, these differences are not enough to account for the big difference in the death rate. The clinical form that coronary heart disease takes also differs between the sexes. Sudden death as the first and only manifestation of the disease is uncommon in women, while angina is fairly often seen; the reverse holds for men. However, an acute heart attack, myocardial infarction, is as likely to prove fatal in women as in men.

The advantage of being female is almost certainly something to do with hormones though precisely what the connection is is not known. Men and women differ in their hormone profiles and the hormonal balance of both changes with age, quite dramatically in the female as she passes through the menopause. Indeed, there is good evidence that the relative immunity of women wears off thereafter, whether the menopause occurs naturally or is artifically induced. In England and Wales the ratio of male to female death rates shows an abrupt change at ages 45-49 years (Figure 9), which would be consistent with a sharp increase in risk affecting post-menopausal women. In one Swedish study it was claimed that women who had ceased menstruating were more liable to develop coronary heart disease than women of the same age who were still menstruating. It has been repeatedly shown that blood

Fig. 9.   Ratio of male to female death rates from coronary heart disease in five-year age-groups from 25–79 years in England and Wales, 1970–72.

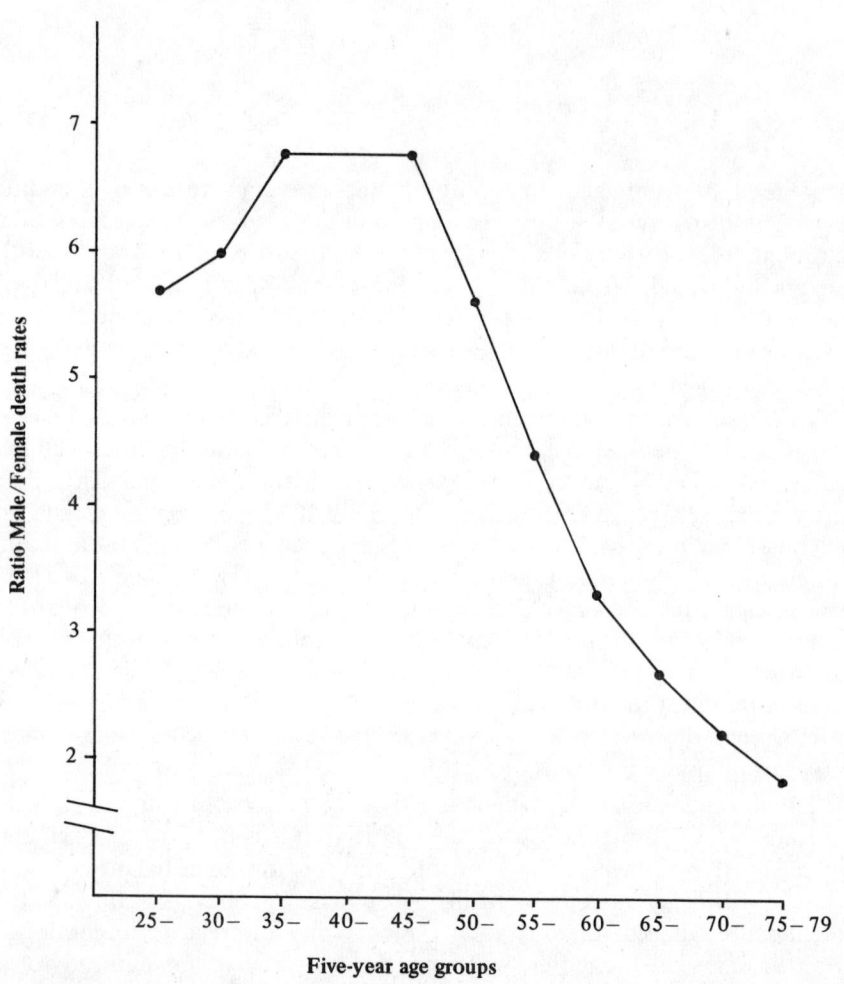

cholesterol is on average higher among women once they have passed the menopause.

But this advantage of being female is being eroded, at least at younger ages. Since the mid-1950s the death rate among females has increased in several countries. While this disturbing trend has been most noticeable among

Fig. 10.   Change in death rates of females from coronary heart
disease in England and Wales, Scotland and Northern Ireland at ages
35–64 years between 1952–56 (A), 1962–66 (B) and 1972–76 (C).

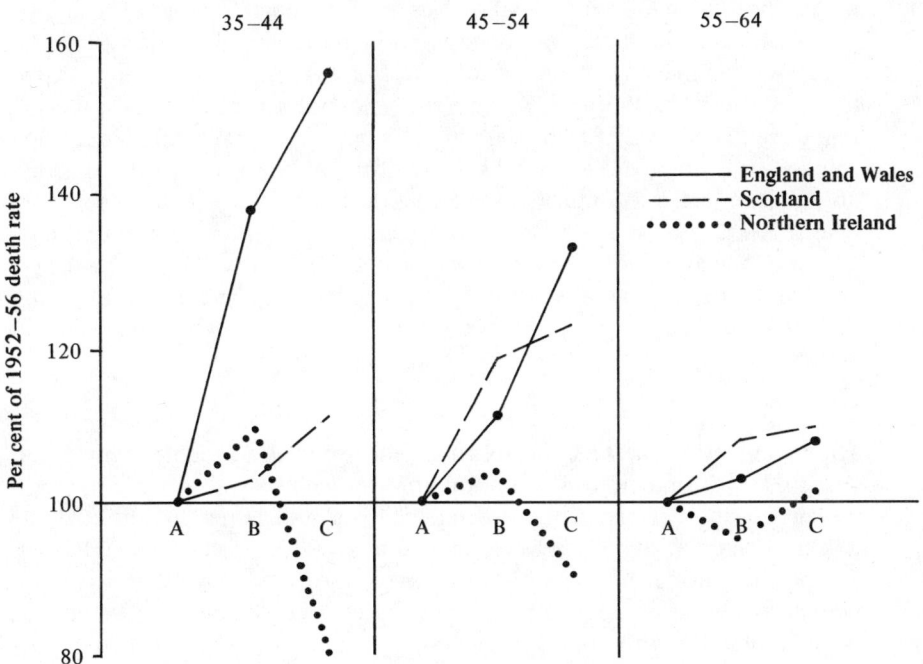

women in their late 30s and early 40s in England and Wales (Figure 10), the
death rate of older women too has shown an upward trend, though not so
marked. In Scotland the same tendencies have been less evident, perhaps
because the rates were initially higher than those in England and Wales. It
would appear that these trends do not apply in Northern Ireland but the data
there are based on much smaller numbers and so must be regarded with
caution. Meanwhile, surveys from various parts of the world show that the
incidence of heart attacks, as well as the death rate, has been increasing in
recent years for women aged 35 and over.

Two factors are thought to account for this rise in the incidence of heart
disease and the death rate and both could be affecting some women
simultaneously. The first and by far the most important is cigarette smoking
and the second, playing a minor role, is the contraceptive pill.

Cigarette smoking

Cigarette smoking has been shown in a number of studies to be a potent risk factor for women as well as for men (see Chapter V). The evidence suggests that women who give up smoking stand to benefit just as much as men; that is, they come to be at lower risk than women who continue to smoke. The highest death rate among females of any population in the world is said to be that of Maori women in New Zealand, and they have the reputation of being also the heaviest smokers. In the UK the proportion of women who smoke has remained fairly steady for the past 20 years or more, but recently the amount smoked on average by each woman who does smoke has increased considerably. It is reported from the United States that sudden death due to coronary heart disease is on the increase among females, and this is attributed to an increase in heavy smoking among women. Some reports suggest that heavy smoking brings on an early menopause; if this is confirmed, it would imply that the biological advantage of pre-menopausal women would disappear at an earlier age.

The contraceptive pill

The introduction of the contraceptive pill provided a reliable, simple and acceptable method of contraception for women. Indeed this method still remains the most effective of those that are reversible. However, although the risks associated with its use are very small indeed, the contraceptive pill is not completely without hazard. Although the risk of coronary heart disease in women is low in comparison with men several studies have indicated that women over 35 on the pill have a slightly increased risk of coronary heart disease when compared with women of the same age not using the pill. Two large studies in this country have reported the outcome of several years' follow-up of some 63,000 women of whom half were on the pill and half not. Despite the large scale of these studies, there were only a score or so of deaths from the disease on which to base the statistical analysis, because coronary heart disease is comparatively rare among young women. So the size of the risk has to be kept in proportion and occurs only among a tiny minority of pill-users. Studies have shown that:

> *in women under 35 the increased risk for those on the pill is so small as to be almost negligible in view of the rarity of the disease in this age group;*
>
> *there is a slightly increased risk for women over 35 on the pill compared with those not on the pill;*
>
> *smokers in the latter group are at rather greater risk.*

The last fact is borne out by all the studies to date that have looked at the point and is, evidently, highly relevant to what has been happening to the death rate of women in this and other countries during the last few years. In 1964 there were about half a million women on the pill in this country; by 1977 the number had increased to more than three million. Over the same period the number of women in the 'packet of cigarettes a day' class had also increased steadily.

The evidence on the possible risks of the contraceptive pill must be viewed with some reservations. In the first place there is not one pill but many different types and these have been changing over the years. It cannot be said for sure as yet that the adverse effects associated with the contraceptive pills that contained relatively large amounts of oestrogen and which were used in the early days of oral contraception, will continue to be seen with the pills containing much lower amounts in use today. Secondly, pill-users are a selected group and other factors quite apart from their use of the pill could be relevant to their risk of coronary heart disease. Thus, they might be subject to greater stress than the non-user, they might be on other medication, they might possibly drink more than other women and so on.

It is important to discuss with the doctor the most appropriate and suitable form of contraception. The decision about what form of contraception to use must be considered in the light of other risk factors and if it is decided that oral contraception is suitable then it is important to pay particular attention to advice about the increased risk of coronary heart disease associated with smoking.

CHAPTER X Father of the man

Inherited characteristics

One of the surest ways of living to a ripe old age is to have parents who have done just that. Conversely, coronary heart disease often seems to run in a family. Patients who suffer from it often give a history of near relatives with the disease. This could be because members of the same family share, to a greater extent than unrelated people, the same 'gene' which determines the characteristics they inherit from their parents. But we do not select our parents. They are given to us and they give us our genes. However, there is no gene for coronary heart disease as such and it cannot be regarded as a purely inherited disease.

This does not mean that genes are irrelevant to coronary heart disease. There are some hints that they do influence a person's susceptibility. The most obvious influence is of course that of a person's sex which is determined by a special component of the genetic make-up of every one of us. The striking differences between men and women in their death rate from this disease have been referred to in Chapter IX.

Genes may be involved in other ways too. There is a rare inherited disease in which, because of a fault, it is thought, in a single gene, the body is unable to handle cholesterol in the normal way, with the result that the blood cholesterol is very high. Unless patients are treated successfully they develop severely diseased patches in the coronary arteries (atheroma) at an early age and may die of coronary heart disease while still in their teens. But if a single abnormal gene can cause this extreme condition, it is reasonable to suppose that the manner in which other related genes behave may explain, at least in part, the variation among seemingly normal people in their blood cholesterol; and that variation, as we say in Chapter VII, is one of the main risk factors for the disease.

One further hint comes from investigations into the frequency of coronary heart disease among twins. A Swedish study of twins in which one or both were affected by the disease revealed that both twins suffered from the disease more often if they were identical twins (and therefore had exactly the same genes) than if they were non-identical twins (and therefore differed to some extent in genetic make-up).

Recent national and international comparisons have suggested that the incidence of coronary heart disease is related to the frequency of different blood groups in the population; people with blood group O may, it appears, be slightly more liable to the disease than those with other blood groups. These findings are not beyond dispute, however, and even if accepted at their face value, the difference in risk between the blood groups is relatively minor. Their interest lies rather in the hint that the blood groups may be signalling the existence of some other as yet unidentified genes or gene groups with an effect on heart disease.

Environment and upbringing

The fact that coronary heart disease can run in the family may be due to inherited characteristics but it could just as easily be because the family shares the same environment and upbringing. Parents do more than bequeath their genes to their offspring — they (usually) bring them up. As everyone knows, children are powerfully influenced in their attitudes and behaviour by their parents ('He's acting just like his father'). Many of these habits and attitudes are directly relevant to the child's susceptibility to coronary heart disease when he or she grows up. Smoking is an obvious instance. Surveys have clearly shown that young people are more likely to be smokers if their parents smoke, and especially if both parents smoke. Dietary habits, likes and dislikes, are also established, in the main, early in life and these too can affect the future chances of coronary heart disease. Thus, obesity in childhood is thought very often to be the forerunner of obesity in later life, and that in turn may predispose to raised blood pressure. According to some doctors childhood obesity can lead to a tendency to one form of diabetes in middle age and that, too, carries an increased risk of coronary heart disease. Too much salt in the diet in infancy and childhood may tend (see Chapter VII) to raise the blood pressure and that raised pressure may then persist as the child grows up. Children are naturally active but the TV set may all too easily convert them to a sedentary lifestyle. Parents should encourage physical activity in the form of outings, hikes, sports and the like; the active child is more likely to become the active adult and another risk factor will have been avoided.

Further evidence of the importance of patterns of behaviour traceable back to a person's early years is to be found in the experience of people who migrate from one country where the rate of coronary heart disease is low to another where the rate is high. The younger the migrant the more likely he is to acquire the habits and mode of life of his adopted country, and the older he is when he leaves his homeland the more he tends to retain the ways of life characteristic of the land of his birth. Not unexpectedly, therefore, it turns out that the younger the immigrant when he migrates to a *high-risk* country, the higher his chances of coronary heart disease later on. This fact has been noted for migrants to Australia from Italy, and to the United States from Japan and from some European countries.

But whether or not coronary heart disease is 'in the family' there is evidence that the disease begins to develop at an early age although the individual may not show any obvious effects of this. Although in rare cases heredity may play a significant role in the development of coronary heart disease, for the most part the mode of life and habits of the individual determine the development of the disease and the extent to which the disease affects the life of the individual. It is all the more important for those with a family record of coronary heart disease to pay careful attention to other risk factors and to exercise this care from childhood.

CHAPTER XI Stress and personality

In previous chapters we have examined a number of possible risk factors for coronary heart disease. In particular, we have singled out smoking, high blood pressure and high blood cholesterol concentration as being independent risk factors. That is to say, whenever it has been possible to disentangle their inter-relationships, it seems that any one of these factors on its own puts one at a greater risk of coronary heart disease. These three factors have proved to be the best predictors of future heart attacks. However when the results of five prospective studies in the United States were pooled, they showed that only 40% of those 40 year old men in the highest category, according to smoking habits, blood pressure and cholesterol level, had a heart attack before the age of 65 and 6% of those in the lowest risk category also suffered such attacks.

These results show how much more likely a heart attack is for the person who smokes, has high blood pressure or high blood cholesterol. But they do not tell the whole story. Indeed they pose further questions. Why did 60% of men at the highest risk not get a heart attack and 6% of men with the lowest risk get one? There may be explanations for this in the design of the experiments (for example, men who smoked at the start of the trial may have given up smoking halfway through the trial period), or in the other, less certain, risk factors discussed in earlier chapters. But there may be other, less tangible, risk factors which have not yet been discussed. In this chapter two such possible risk factors are considered: stress and personality.

Stress
Everyone thinks they know what stress is even if they might be hard pressed to define it; and despite attempts to do so no one has come forward with an acceptable way of measuring stress.

The heart and the circulatory system certainly respond to stress; the pulse rate quickens, the skin blood vessels contract (making more blood available for the muscles' immediate use), the blood pressure rises, and so on. (During a race the pulse rate of a racing driver may momentarily jump up to 3 times the rate at rest). These are normal reactions; they are the signals to indicate that the body is getting ready for 'fight or flight'. The question is whether these normal reflexes can somehow lead to disease—may they, for instance, cause persistently raised blood pressure—because the responses have been invoked too often or for too long without relaxation.

Stress can take many forms. One thing that puts a strain on people is finding themselves in an unfamiliar environment where everything and everybody can seem to be vaguely hostile and threatening. In some studies it has been noted that men who change jobs frequently are more prone to coronary heart disease than their contemporaries who stay in the same job. Men who move from one area to another have been found to be at greater risk than men who do not do so. In several separate studies in the United States it was found that men who moved from rural areas to work in large cities were three or four times more liable to get a coronary than those who had stayed home on the farm. In some of these studies it was claimed that the effect of differences in diet, smoking habits, blood pressure and relative weight could all be discounted as explanations for the difference in death rate. Another form of unfamiliar environment is that encountered by people who 'move up in the world', particularly if the individual is unprepared for what he has to contend with in his new social or professional milieu. Some American studies have linked these changes in social status with an increased incidence of coronary heart disease.

Stress cannot be associated with a particular job or way of life but only with the way in which an individual responds to it.

As well as mobility in its various forms—occupational, geographical, social—the misfortunes that befall people on life's way cause stress. A sudden bereavement or loss of one's job are examples of upheavals which are likely to cause stress and it has been reported that men who have had to face shocks of this kind tend to have more heart attacks than would be expected otherwise amongst men of their age. The fascinating aspect of the whole question of stress, however, is how some people seem able to take in their stride 'the slings and arrows of outrageous fortune' while others are unable to cope with relatively minor buffetings. The differences between people in their response to life's challenges could be the missing dimension in the risk factors for coronary heart disease.

Personality

It is sometimes said that it is easy to spot the sort of individual who is going to get a coronary; and over the past two decades or so a start has been made in laying a scientific foundation for this intuitive recognition of the coronary-prone personality. The work originated in America where psychologists studied the characteristics of patients with coronary heart disease and compared them with those of people without the disease. These studies led them to define what became known as the Type A personality, reflecting those traits which the coronary patients displayed more often than the others. The original work has since been confirmed by researchers in Australia, Israel, the Netherlands, Sweden and the UK, which certainly suggests that a type of personality really exists with a special liability to the disease. In general these studies have involved patients who have already had one or more attacks of heart disease, so the studies are open to the objection that the personality traits are the result rather than the cause of the disease. However, there is at least one propective study reported in which apparently healthy middle aged men were initially classified as either possessing or not possessing a Type A personality. It became evident after four years that the Type A men were developing the disease more often than the others; and after eight years it was claimed that the disease occurred twice as often among the Type A men, even allowing for the usual risk factors of smoking, high blood pressure, raised blood cholesterol concentration, and relative weight.

Characteristically, Type A people are strivers, ambitious and competitive. They are impatient and always seem pressed for time. They may often be so acutely aware that time is precious that they can tell you the time correct to within a few minutes without looking at a watch! They eat fast and talk fast. In conversation they will interrupt and finish your sentence for you if you hesitate for a word. They constantly give the impression of trying to do too many things at once. As you would expect, they tend to move job or home more often than non-A people.

When we seek to classify people by their traits we are not measuring them anything like as precisely as when we record blood pressure or cholesterol concentrations. It is all the more remarkable therefore that a rough and ready classification—and that is what Type A really is—should be related so consistently to coronary heart disease. A variety of possible body mechanisms have been suggested which could provide the bridge between personality and coronary heart disease but firm evidence is not yet available as to the nature of the link.

However it can be seen that stress and personality are closely linked as risk factors in coronary heart disease and avoidance of stressful situations is more important to some than to others. Relaxation after stress may be achieved by people in many different ways, it is not only that some people, more than others, take stress in their stride—it is a fact that they appear to thrive on it and are never happier than when under pressure. And for most, if not all, some degree of stress, either permanent or intermittent, connected with work or private lives, is an unavoidable part of life itself. If indeed such stress may be harmful, at least for some, then the best advice may well be to make sure of relaxation, whether reading, listening to the radio or record player, or simply walking the dog and enjoying the open air.

Hobbies, sport and other interests away from everyday work are ways in which the anxieties and tensions of life may be forgotten and those who cannot easily relax may find such diversions more acceptable and more successful in countering the ill-effects of stress and, perhaps, their own personality.

CHAPTER XII Summing up

Chapter I started with the sad story of J B Smith, the salesman from Liverpool who died of a heart attack. The details were disguised but it was a true story. In successive chapters the risk factors which increase the likelihood of contracting coronary heart disease have been discussed and it is clear that whilst we do not fully understand the causes of coronary heart disease we do know how to reduce considerably the risk of developing it.

Coronary heart disease kills and disables many thousands of people every year in this country alone. In 1978, 184,819 people died of coronary heart disease in the UK; 28% of all deaths that year were due to the disease. Many more suffered from angina or other disabling effects of heart attacks. Much of this suffering is avoidable if the advice in this book is followed. It is never too late to change your habits — those who have already survived a heart attack will benefit too.

Smoking is, on the evidence we have, clearly the biggest known risk factor. A man aged 50 who smokes more than 20 cigarettes a day is four times more likely to develop coronary heart disease than a non-smoker of the same age. Smoking also increases the risk for women, particularly if they are taking oral contraceptives when over 35 years old. Giving up smoking is not easy but those who do so not only greatly reduce the risk of dying from a heart attack (see Chapter V) but are also less likely to develop such diseases as chronic bronchitis and lung cancer.

Raised blood pressure is also an important risk factor. There are very effective treatments but it is most important to follow your doctor's advice carefully.

Diet matters. There are benefits to be gained by reducing the proportion of fat in the diet. The reduction in energy intake which results from eating less fat can be made up by eating more bread and more fresh fruit and vegetables including potatoes. Table 2 on page 41 gives a guide to desirable weights for adults and one should always aim to keep within the range for one's height. For most people the message is to eat — and drink — in moderation.

Exercise and relaxation are important and can usefully be combined. The thing to do is to find an activity you enjoy, which takes your mind off the cares of everyday life and, preferably, involves some physical exertion.

In Chapter X the influence of inherited characteristics and of environment was discussed. It may be that some people have something in their genetic make-up which causes them to be more susceptible to coronary heart disease. Attitudes and patterns of behaviour appear to be learnt to some extent from our parents; for example, the children of smokers are more likely to smoke than the children of non-smokers. Thus people whose relatives suffer from coronary heart disease need to take special care.

Plan to avoid a heart attack

There are a few simple rules. They cannot guarantee you freedom from coronary heart disease but if you follow them you will substantially increase your chances of enjoying a longer healthier life. Prevention is better than cure. It is no good waiting until coronary heart disease restricts your activities; heart surgery is expensive and can help only a few.

The rules are:

1. DON'T SMOKE;

2. If you have high blood pressure pay special attention to your doctor's advice;

3. Maintain ideal weight;

4. Be careful about the amount of fat you eat;

5. Find a way of relaxing which you enjoy, preferably a way which involves some exertion.

Glossary

Angina (pectoris)	—	a chest pain, often, though not always, due to coronary heart disease.
Atheroma	—	a condition in which deposits build up in the inner lining of major arteries.
Calorie	—	unit for measuring energy.
Cholesterol	—	a fat-like substance found normally in many body tissues, including the blood.
Coronary artery	—	an artery supplying the heart with blood.
Coronary heart disease	—	result of damaged coronary arteries; can take three main forms—sudden death, myocardial infarction, and angina pectoris.
Coronary thrombosis	—	a blockage in a coronary artery caused by the formation of a blood clot.
Electrocardiograph	—	an instrument which measures the changes in electrical activity in the heart during the contraction cycle.
Gene	—	a unit in heredity, usually regarded as controlling a single trait.
Haemoglobin	—	the substance in the red blood cells which links up with and transports oxygen.
Hypertension	—	an abnormally high blood pressure.
Incidence	—	the number of new events in a stated period related to the size of the population; eg 45 coronary attacks per 1000 population per annum.

Infarct — a portion of tissue that has died as the result of an interruption of its blood supply.

Intervention study — an investigation in which an attempt is made to change the characteristics of a group of individuals and to measure subsequent effects on the incidence of disease.

Ischaemic heart disease — a disease of the heart in which there is an insufficient blood supply to the myocardium (see fig. 1), usually due to disease of the coronary arteries.

Myocardial infarction — a form of coronary heart disease, which may or may not be fatal, in which a section of the myocardium is damaged because the blood supply is cut off.

Myocardium — the muscle of the heart.

Oestrogen — a female sex hormone.

Prevalence — number of cases in existence at a given moment related to the size of the population.

Prospective study — an investigation in which the attributes of each individual in a group are noted and the subsequent history of each one is followed over a period.

Retrospective study — an investigation of a group of people who already possess an attribute (eg a disease) to see what factors may have caused it.

Risk factor — anything which puts a person at a higher than average risk of something (eg a disease) happening to him or her.

Standardised death rate — a death rate that has been adjusted for age, and also sometimes for sex, in such a way as to allow direct comparisons between populations that differ in their age (and sex) composition.

Standardised mortality ratio — the number of deaths occurring in a population divided by the number that would have been expected to occur under standard conditions, usually expressed as a percentage.

A short list for further reading

Detailed references to the large — and expanding — technical literature on coronary heart disease would have been out of place in the present document. For the non-technical reader interested in pursuing the subject the following books may prove of help: each has a list of references to medical and other journals:-

British Regional Heart Study: geographic variations in cardiovascular mortality, and the role of water quality — S J Pocock, A G Shaper, D G Cook, R F Packham, R F Lacey, P Powell, P F Russell (British Medical Journal, 24 May 1980).

Contrasting Concepts of Ischaemic Heart Disease — G Biorck (the 1974 Lilly Lectures given at Oxford and London).

Diet and Coronary Heart Disease — HMSO 1974 (report by an independent group of experts advising the Government).

Eating for Health — HMSO 1978 (deals generally with preventive aspects of diet and nutrition, with references to coronary heart disease).

Health Services in Scotland: Report for 1975 — HMSO 1976 (contains a summary of the 'water connection').

Prevention of Coronary Heart Disease — Royal College of Physicians, 1976 (report of a joint working party of the Royal College of Physicians of London and the British Cardiac Society).

The Enigma of Coronary Heart Disease — A H T Robb-Smith, 1967 (a pathologist examines the question: 'Is it a new disease?').

Uses of Epidemiology — J N Morris. 3rd edition, 1975 (a general text but with many references to coronary heart disease).

Leaflets on smoking, nutrition, exercise and fitness are available free from the Health Education Council (78 New Oxford St, London WC1). For people living in Scotland, leaflets on many of the subjects covered in this booklet can be obtained free from the Scottish Health Education Group (Woodburn

House, Canaan Lane, Edinburgh EH10 4FG). In addition, leaflets on methods of contraception are available free from the Family Planning Information Service (27−35 Waterman St, London W1).

Printed in England for Her Majesty's Stationery Office by Commercial Colour Press, London E.7.
Dd.717236 C600 10/81